W9-BYM-158

Understanding Your Food
Allergies and Intolerances

Trusted Advice for a Healthier Life
from Harvard Medical School

Understanding Your Food Allergies and Intolerances

A Guide to Management and Treatment

Wayne G. Shreffler, MD,
and Qian Yuan, MD
with Karen Asp

St. Martin's Paperbacks

NOTE: If you purchased this book without a cover you should be aware that this book is stolen property. It was reported as "unsold and destroyed" to the publisher, and neither the author nor the publisher has received any payment for this "stripped book."

The information in this book is not intended to replace the advice of the reader's own physician or other medical professional. You should consult a medical professional in matters relating to health, especially if you have existing medical conditions, and before starting, stopping or changing the dose of any medication you are taking. Individual readers are solely responsible for their own health-care decisions. The author and the publisher do not accept responsibility for any adverse effects individuals may claim to experience, whether directly or indirectly, from the information contained in this book.

The fact that an organization or Web site is mentioned in the book as a potential source of information does not mean that the author or the publisher endorses any of the information it may provide or recommendations it may make.

The stories in this book are composite, fictional accounts based on the experiences of many individuals. Similarities to any real person or persons are coincidental and unintentional.

UNDERSTANDING YOUR FOOD ALLERGIES AND INTOLERANCES

Copyright © 2012 by Harvard University.

All rights reserved.

For information address St. Martin's Press, 175 Fifth Avenue, New York, NY 10010.

EAN: 978-0-312-55332-6

Printed in the United States of America

St. Martin's Paperbacks edition / June 2012

St. Martin's Paperbacks are published by St. Martin's Press, 175 Fifth Avenue, New York, NY 10010.

10 9 8 7 6 5 4 3 2 1

To my wife, Annie, and children, Addy and Katie
　　　　　　　　　　—FROM WAYNE

To my wife, Weimeng (Theresa), and children,
Melissa and Mariel-Lulu
　　　　　　　　　　—FROM QIAN

To my husband, Chris Pataluch
　　　　　　　　　　—FROM KAREN

contents

part I

Understanding Food Sensitivities

chapter 1

Learning the Lingo

Have you ever eaten a certain food (or foods) and then felt sick a few minutes or even a few hours later? Maybe you got an itchy mouth, felt nauseous, or had diarrhea. Or perhaps you've noticed that you simply feel better if you avoid certain foods. If so, you could be one of millions of Americans with a food sensitivity.

There are two types of food sensitivities—food allergies and food intolerances—and because they share some characteristics, they're often confused. So how do you know which one you have? Unfortunately, that's not an easy question to answer, especially because there's so much confusion about food sensitivities in general. Food sensitivities even baffle doctors!

It's tough to understand, after all, why food might be an enemy when your body needs food to exist. To quote the Roman poet and philosopher Lucretius, "What is food to one man may be fierce poison to others." So what is it about certain foods that upset the body, and why does it only happen to a select group of individuals?

If you're reading this book, you've probably asked these same questions. Perhaps you or someone you know suffers from a food sensitivity. While we can't provide definitive answers to all of your questions—unfortunately, there's a lot that's still unknown about food sensitivities—we will share our combined expertise and give you the information you need to manage and treat your condition.

Because let's face it: One of the greatest joys in life is eating. Think how many times, after all, you've gathered around a table of food with friends and family to celebrate an event, mark a special occasion, or just enjoy each other's company. Imagine what those events would be like without food. Perhaps not as enjoyable, right?

Yet if you have a food sensitivity, that joy of eating can be significantly reduced, as you live in constant fear that you might eat a food that makes you sick. You may no longer enjoy going out to eat, whether to a restaurant or somebody else's house, and because you're always having to pick apart food labels, shopping for foods has become a major burden. There's also a chance that if you've cut many foods from your diet, you may be falling short on some nutrients, which could set you up for other health problems. Plain and simple, when you have a food sensitivity, finding the joy in eating is much more of a challenge.

Fortunately, though, you don't have to be defeated. Granted, if you have a food sensitivity, you will have to be more diligent about what you eat, which means life may be a little tougher. Yet here's the good news: A food sensitivity doesn't have to stop you from enjoying life. With this book as your guide, you can learn how to manage your food sensitivity and reap the rewards—both emotionally and physically—that food offers.

What Is—and What Isn't—a Food Sensitivity?

Pardon the pun, but food sensitivities aren't easy to digest. That's because when it comes to food sensitivities, there's no clear-cut definition. The medical community doesn't even agree on a definition for "food sensitivity." The term has also been skewed in the minds of consumers, for what you call a food sensitivity may be entirely different from what your friend calls a food sensitivity.

To help avoid this confusion, we're going to use one simple definition for "food sensitivity" throughout this book: a reproducible, adverse reaction to a food.

As you can see, "food sensitivity" is an umbrella term for many but not all adverse reactions to food. Reproducibility is crucial to our definition of food sensitivities, for while food poisoning is also an adverse reaction to food, it's generally not reproducible. In other words, you could eat the same type of food (but not the exact food per se) again, and as long as it wasn't contaminated with toxins or bacteria, you would be okay. Thus, food poisoning doesn't meet our definition of food sensitivity, which is why we won't be covering that topic in this book.

What we will be covering, though, are two sensitivities that often get confused: food intolerances and food allergies. Both are reproducible adverse reactions to food, and while they do have overlapping characteristics, there are important differences between the two.

By the way, both of us see patients with allergies in our offices, but our focus is slightly different. Dr. Wayne sees mainly children who are struggling with what we call immediate allergies, which you'll learn about later in this chapter. Dr. Qian, on the other hand, focuses on the gastrointestinal aspect of food allergies. We also see patients together in a multidisciplinary clinic focused on eosinophilic gastrointestinal disease, which we'll discuss later in this book.

Intolerance Versus Allergy—
Setting the Record Straight

Before we start distinguishing the differences between food intolerance and food allergy, we'd like you to meet two women who represent typical patients in our offices. Each woman complained about adverse reactions to food, but, as you'll see, the diagnosis for each one was quite different.

Kathy's Story

Kathy was in her early forties when she began to experience nagging stomach issues, especially within hours of eating particular foods. She would get bloated and have cramping abdominal pain and excess gas (but no itching, swelling, congestion, or wheezing). She also suffered from periodic headaches, fatigue, and an occasional bout of diarrhea brought on for no apparent reason. The symptoms would get progressively worse for about a week or two, and then they'd gradually diminish.

Over time, Kathy began to see a pattern: Every time she ate pasta or bread, she felt sick, which led her to suspect that wheat was the culprit behind her symptoms. So she began cutting some wheat- and gluten-based foods from her diet. Over time, she began to feel better, and the annoying stomach problems she used to get gradually improved.

Yet she was never entirely symptom-free. She continued to have abdominal pain, bloating, gassiness, and diarrhea, which led her to believe she might have a food allergy. Throughout the years, Kathy had seen several doctors, including allergists, but each time she went, no doctor could find anything wrong with her.

So at fifty years old, she sought help from a gastroenterologist for another set of tests, including blood tests; an upper endoscopy, a procedure that allows the gastroenterologist to examine the esophagus, stomach, and small bowel through a thin, flexible tube; and a colonoscopy. While the blood test checked for food allergies and the colonoscopy looked for evidence of inflammation of the colon, which could indicate a few different health conditions, the upper endoscopy was looking for a condition called celiac disease. All the test results, though, came back normal.

As a result, the doctor could tell her what she didn't have—she had neither a food allergy nor celiac disease—but he couldn't confirm what she did have. He could only assume that because she appeared to get better when she cut wheat from her diet, she must have an intolerance to wheat. The solution? Avoid foods and food products that contain wheat.

Since then, Kathy adjusted her diet so she doesn't consume wheat. She's had to be more careful about reading food labels and choosing restaurants that can cater to her needs, but all of her diligence has paid off. Food no longer makes her sick. Sure, there are those rare occasions when she's accidentally eaten wheat and suffered a few minor stomach woes as a result, but they haven't lasted more than a day. Kathy's hopeful that in the future, she can eat wheat again—she's heard, after all, that you can outgrow your intolerances—but until then, she'll just watch her diet.

Jennifer's Story

Jennifer, on the other hand, was thirty-two when she had her first reaction to shrimp. She'd suffered from seasonal allergies ever since she was in high school—spring has always been her worst season—but food had never given her any problems. Plus, she'd occasionally eaten shrimp throughout the years, especially during vacations to the beach. She remembers having some stomach cramps one time years ago after eating shrimp, but it wasn't enough to cause any major alarms. At the time, she thought maybe the shrimp just wasn't fresh.

Yet when she attended a friend's party and ate a shrimp appetizer, she broke out in hives and began to have difficulty breathing. Her husband whisked her to the emergency room, where she was given an injection of epinephrine, a medication that treats severe allergic reactions; Benadryl; and a dose of steroids.

When she later saw an allergist, she tested positive for shellfish allergy. Jennifer has since had to give up eating all shellfish and must take extra precautions to avoid contact with shellfish and foods that might be contaminated with shellfish. That often means taking special precautions at restaurants, informing friends who invite her to dinner, and being extra careful about grocery shopping.

Because allergies like this can cause a severe allergic reaction called anaphylaxis, Jennifer also carries epinephrine wherever she goes. She's never had to use the epinephrine, but she and her husband know how to use it in case she does accidentally eat or come in contact with shrimp. For Jennifer, this will probably be a life-long problem.

How Your Immune System Determines the Difference Between Food Intolerances and Food Allergies

It's true that food was making both Kathy and Jennifer sick. Yet their symptoms and treatment plans were different. In Jennifer's case, a food allergy, a disease that's well understood by the medical community and has been widely studied, was the root of her problems.

Yet Kathy's experience was entirely different. Because tests ruled out food allergy and there are few tests to diagnose a food intolerance, the doctor had to conclude that Kathy was suffering from an intolerance, which, with some exceptions, is not a well-defined disease.

Of course, that still doesn't answer one big question: What's the difference between a food intolerance and a food allergy? To help clear up the confusion, take a look at how we're defining these two conditions:

- **Food intolerance**: a reproducible, adverse reaction to a food that's not the direct result of an immune response
- **Food allergy**: a reproducible, adverse reaction to a food that's caused by a type of immune reaction to a food protein

Note the main difference between those two definitions: the role of the immune system, your body's defense mechanism that protects you against germs, diseases, and other foreign invaders. Food intolerances by definition are not directly caused by an immune response to a food protein, while food allergies are, and that's the main difference between the two. Allergists actually think about food in a specific way when trying to understand whether an individual's symptoms are caused by an allergy. Simply put, they think about the protein of the food.

Most foods, including fruits and vegetables, which aren't usually major sources of proteins nutritionally, contain proteins (or allergens, as we'll call them) that may be recognized by your immune system as foreign. On the other hand, some things you eat, like pure fats or sugars, don't contain significant amounts of allergens. That's why if somebody tells an allergist that he or she may be allergic to corn because symptoms manifest after eating high-fructose corn syrup, the allergist suspects there's probably another explanation for the symptoms. Perhaps the person can't absorb large amounts of fructose (which indicates an intolerance) or could be having problems because of another ingredient.

There is one condition, though, celiac disease, that's a little trickier to classify because, in it, the immune system does play a central role. However, most physicians don't classify celiac disease as an allergy since the disease is actually a response of the immune system to proteins in the body versus those in food. Essentially, the immune system begins attacking itself, and although the attack is triggered by exposure to gluten, the damaging response is directed at proteins in the body, not those in gluten. We'll discuss celiac disease in greater detail in a later chapter about food intolerances.

The Skinny on Food Intolerances

Kathy isn't alone in suspecting she had a food allergy. Because symptoms of food allergies and food intolerances often overlap, many people think they have a food allergy when they actually have a food intolerance. In fact, you can have intolerances to multiple foods, which is why it can be tough to figure out exactly what food is causing your problems. The most common intolerances, though, are to wheat and other gluten-containing grains, sugar found in fruits and honey, cow's milk and dairy products, and corn products, according to the American Gastroenterological Association.

So what causes food intolerances? Some intolerances, like lactose, fructose, and sucrose intolerances, are due to a lack of specific digestive enzymes in the gastrointestinal tract. Other causes of intolerances remain a mystery.

Symptoms typically occur within hours after eating the food. The severity of these symptoms may also depend on the amount of the offending food you've eaten, especially when it comes to lactose intolerance. The more lactose you've consumed, the worse your symptoms may be.

To make matters more confusing, you don't always have the same reaction to the same food. While you might have excess gas one time, you could have cramping another time.

Unfortunately, though, with the exceptions of intolerances to lactose, fructose, and sucrose and of celiac disease, food intolerances are difficult to diagnose definitively. In fact, tests for most food intolerances don't exist. Often, the only way to diagnose your condition is by going on an elimination diet, where you completely avoid the suspected offending foods. If you feel better, that suggests you have an intolerance to that food. If you want to confirm your findings, you may try reintroducing the food or keeping a diary of symptoms and the foods you're eating. (See "Starting a Food Diary" for more information.)

The best news about food intolerances? With the exception of celiac disease, they aren't associated with long-term or severe health consequences. Even better, for many individuals, intolerances may be temporary. This may be because they're secondary to another problem (for instance, lactose intolerance during a gastrointestinal

Starting a Food Diary

If you've ever tried to lose weight, you're probably familiar with the concept of a food diary where you write down everything you eat and drink. We sometimes use the same thing with food sensitivities, and we recommend that you keep one to help you or your doctor figure out if you have a food sensitivity and, if so, what type you have.

In your food diary, write down everything you eat and drink in a day's time. Then record any negative reactions you suspect you've had to food. You can also answer the following questions about each reaction (these, by the way, are the same questions a doctor will ask you):

- How quickly after eating did your suspected reaction occur?
- Did you take any medicines like antihistamines to make you feel better? If so, did they help?
- Is your suspected reaction always associated with a certain food?
- Can you sometimes eat that food without experiencing any reaction?
- Did other people who ate the same food feel sick?
- How much did you eat before you had a reaction?

(continued)

- Were you eating other foods at the same time you had
  the reaction?

  If you do seek medical help, bring your food diary with
  you, since it can be an invaluable tool in helping your doctor
  diagnose your condition.

infection) or related to maturation (for example, many
toddlers may develop a greater capacity to absorb fructose with age).

Getting to Know Food Allergies

Food allergies, on the other hand, are generally more
severe than intolerances, either because they can be immediately life-threatening or because they may be more
strongly associated with inflammation of the gastrointestinal tract, which can lead to more serious long-term
consequences. As you can see in the above scenarios, if
Kathy were to eat a small amount of wheat, her symptoms would clear up in a day or so. Yet if Jennifer were
to eat any shrimp, her symptoms could be so severe she
might have go to go the emergency room. In rare cases,

food allergies can even be fatal. So what's going on with food allergies?

For the majority of people, eating a food your body doesn't know—and just think how many foreign foods you eat in a lifetime!—doesn't raise any red flags in your immune system. It accepts the food, even if it's never met it before, and life goes on without a hitch. But that's not the case with somebody who has a food allergy.

The immune system of food-allergic individuals views the food as harmful to your body. Although you can develop allergies to any food, about 90 percent of all food allergy reactions are triggered by eight foods: milk, soy, eggs, wheat, peanuts, tree nuts, fish, and shellfish. Most food allergies develop in childhood, but, as in Jennifer's case above, they can occur in adulthood as well.

From what we understand about the immune system, the allergen must have been "seen" by the body in some way before the first allergic reaction. However, allergic reactions can occur with the first known ingestion of a particular food. Case in point: Well over half of young children seen by an allergist for a reaction to peanuts have never eaten them.

As mentioned above, it's the protein, which is composed of molecules made from building blocks called amino acids, in food that triggers a reaction. We call these proteins allergens, and, depending on the food, there are usually only one or a few proteins that are important allergens in each food. These proteins stimulate the immune system, which springs into action to protect you from what it perceives to be a threat. As a result, you develop symptoms.

These symptoms are more serious than those associated with food intolerances and involve more body systems. Symptoms can run the gamut from eczema, itching in the mouth, hives, vomiting, diarrhea, and abdominal pain all the way to anaphylaxis, a severe and sometimes fatal whole-body allergic response that can cause respiratory failure or shock.

Because those symptoms can occur anywhere from minutes to several hours after eating the offending food— even a trace amount of the food can set off a reaction— food allergies are divided into two types: immediate and delayed.

We'll tackle these two types in more detail in chapter 6, but, for now, understand that "immediate" means just what it sounds like: symptoms occur within minutes to hours. Meanwhile, symptoms of delayed food allergies may develop more than a day after eating the offending food protein.

The immune system, after all, has multiple players, and some are associated with more chronic, slowly evolving responses. Some forms of food allergy, espe-

Muscling Through the Myths

Do a search online for "food sensitivities" and thousands of results will pop up, including many myths about food sensitivities. Our patients are always asking us about these myths, which is why we thought it might be interesting to compile a list of the most common ones. Throughout the book, we'll show you why they're not true.

- Because I've had an adverse reaction to food, I must have a food allergy.
- A simple blood test can tell me what food intolerances I have.
- Food allergy equals anaphylaxis.
- Food allergies get increasingly worse with each food exposure.
- A positive allergy-testing result means that I have a definite allergic reaction to a specific food.
- Celiac disease is a food allergy.
- An allergy test can tell me how "allergic" I am.
- Food sensitivities can cause or worsen developmental disorders like autism and Aspberger's syndrome.

cially those that affect the gut, are caused by those slower-responding components. Some people with food allergies can even experience a mix of immediate and delayed immune responses.

Although there are various ways that a food allergy reaction can be treated once an accidental ingestion has occurred, avoiding the offending food is still the main treatment.

chapter 2

Who's Most at Risk for Developing a Food Sensitivity?

We get lots of questions from patients, but some of the toughest to answer are these: Why do I have a food sensitivity? Does it have to do with something in the environment? maybe something I ate as a kid? even my genes?

To all of those questions, we have one answer: maybe. We wish we could tell you why you have a food sensitivity, be it a food intolerance or a food allergy, but because there are so many factors involved, pinpointing exact causes is not only difficult but also usually impossible.

That being said, though, we have identified risk factors for some food sensitivities, including where you live and your ethnicity, your family history, your age, your gender, and certain health conditions. This doesn't mean, however, that we can predict who's going to develop a food sensitivity, but we do have some general ideas about who might be at greater risk.

Unfortunately, though, risk factors for food sensitivities aren't like those for heart disease or diabetes, many of which you can control. For instance, it's well established that a risk factor for cardiovascular disease is being overweight. If you want to decrease your risk for heart disease, you can lose weight by increasing your physical activity levels and following a healthier diet. Not so with food sensitivities.

Risk factors for food sensitivities are largely out of your control. You can't, after all, change your family history any more than you can change your ethnic background. Yet we still think it's important to be aware of these risk factors, especially because our patients ask about them so frequently.

What Your Address and Ethnicity Say About Your Food Sensitivity Risk

As far-fetched as this might sound, your address and ethnic background could play a role in whether you develop a food sensitivity.

Researchers have long known that food allergies in

particular are more prevalent in industrialized nations than in developing countries. Take peanut allergies, for instance. Although Chinese and Americans eat about the same amounts of peanuts, the prevalence of peanut allergy is higher in the United States than in China.

Celiac disease is another condition that plays favorites when it comes to geographic location. While it's prevalent in Europe, North and South America, Australia, North Africa, the Middle East, and south Asia, it rarely occurs in people from other parts of Asia or sub-Saharan Africa.

There are also differences when evaluating ethnicity in food-intolerant individuals. Asians, African Americans, and Hispanics, for instance, have a higher prevalence of lactose intolerance than do other ethnic groups. Asians are also more susceptible to developing alcohol intolerance.

With Age Comes Wisdom—and Fewer Food Allergies?

Here's a good reason not to dread birthdays anymore: with age comes a reduction in your risk for most food allergies. Unfortunately, we can't say the same about food intolerances, which seem to have no age limits and can develop at any age.

Most food allergies actually begin early in life. While it's tough to say exactly what percentage of allergies begin by the age of one, we can say that the majority of children with food allergies outgrow them by the time they're four or five years old. As children age, their symptoms either disappear or, at the very least, diminish. Allergies to milk, soy, wheat, and egg are the ones that usually vanish with age, while allergies to shellfish, peanuts, and tree nuts tend to persist through adulthood.

Why do food allergies develop at a higher rate earlier in life rather than later in life, and what are the risk factors for that occurrence? This is an area of controversy and shifting consensus. Here's one theory: The immaturity of young children's immune systems may make them more prone to allergies.

Yet another theory involves the maturity of the gut. The thought is that children may have a more permeable gastrointestinal tract, and as they digest food, more food allergens may escape the intestinal tract. As a result, those food proteins may become easy targets for the body's immune system. Although this idea hasn't been proved, it probably contributed to the conservative recommendations for introduction of commonly allergenic foods to infants and toddlers that, until recently, medical experts followed for many years.

A contrasting theory emphasizes how much exposure children have had to food allergens. We're beginning to suspect that tolerance of foods is associated with consuming that food regularly. In other words, the more often you eat a certain food, the more accustomed your body becomes to that food, and the less it treats that food as a foreigner. Consequently, by not eating these allergy-prone foods on a regular basis early in life, the rate of allergies may actually be increasing. This concept represents a significant shift in thought from a few years ago. Because an increasing number of studies has failed to show that early avoidance protects from allergy and may actually increase its prevalence, recommendations from multiple professional societies including the American Academy of Pediatrics and the American Academy of Allergy, Asthma and Immunology no longer support early avoidance.

We should mention, though, that while most food allergies develop in childhood, it is possible to develop a food allergy as an adult for no apparent reason. Take, for instance, shellfish (especially crustaceans like shrimp, crab, and lobster) and peanuts and tree nuts, which are the two allergies that most commonly strike adults. Other allergies do also occur—Dr. Wayne once treated a woman who developed a severe immediate food allergy to milk during her first pregnancy even after she had tolerated milk well as a child—but, overall, these are unusual cases, and we often can't explain why a person develops an allergy as an adult.

Two things to note about adults who develop severe food allergies: First, these individuals usually have some other allergy. In fact, it's rare that an individual who's not already allergic to something, be it pollen or another food, will develop a food allergy as an adult. Second, these individuals usually develop allergies to foods they're not eating regularly. Take, for instance, Jennifer, whom you met in chapter 1. Not only did she suffer from seasonal allergies, she also rarely ate shellfish. The combination of those two factors puts her at higher risk of developing a food allergy.

Note, though, that there is one exception to the above discussion regarding one of the most common forms of food allergy in adults: a mild food allergy related primarily to pollen allergens, which we'll discuss in chapter 6.

You Can't Hide from Your Genes— How Family History May Play a Role in Food Sensitivities

You can thank your parents for your height, your eye color, and, yes, even your food sensitivity. Let's look at food allergies first since there's more data to support a genetic link.

Numerous studies have proved that allergies run in families. That's why one of the first questions doctors will often ask you if they suspect a food allergy is whether you have a family history. (That's why it's also a good idea to know your family history of various illnesses and diseases. If you don't know this information, it's time to start asking—quiz your immediate family members to find out what health conditions have affected your parents and siblings.)

So what does having a family history mean? In a nutshell, if you have any family history of atopic disease, essentially any condition in which the body produces an IgE response to external stimuli, you're at increased risk of developing a food allergy. Those atopic diseases include asthma, allergic rhinitis (hay fever), atopic dermatitis (eczema), and food allergies.

Here's how much that family history inflates your risk of any allergic disease, which includes food allergies:

- If you have one parent with some form of allergy, your risk of developing an allergy of any type is 25 percent.
- If both of your parents have some form of allergy, your risk of developing an allergy of any type is at least 50 percent or more.

One of the most convincing arguments about the genetic link in food allergies comes from a well-known study on twins. In this study from the *Journal of Allergy and Clinical Immunology,* identical twins were both peanut-allergic 64 percent of the time, while among non-identical twins, the rate dropped to 7 percent.

Those numbers might sound high, but don't be alarmed. In reality, although food allergy does have a genetic component, genes don't explain the whole story, for not all children in the same family, identical twins included, have food allergies, and when they do, they don't necessarily share the same allergies. While one child might have an allergy to peanuts, another might suffer from hay fever, while the third child is completely allergy-free. The upshot? Although family history increases your risk, family history alone doesn't mean you're destined to develop a food allergy.

Even if you have no first-degree relatives with a history of atopic disease, you can still have allergies, although your risk is much lower. Crazy, yes? Not if you consider the dramatic increase in food allergies in recent years. That increase has happened too rapidly to be explained by genetic changes, which underscores the fact that environmental factors also influence the development of food allergies.

With food intolerances, genetics can also come into play. Take, for instance, lactose intolerance, which has been shown to have a genetic link. It's more prevalent in certain ethnic groups, and Asians, African Americans, and Hispanics tend to develop clinical symptoms of lactose intolerance at a younger age than Caucasians.

Celiac disease is also genetically related. If one family member has celiac disease, screening for all first-degree relatives should be considered, as there's a high likelihood they also have this condition. In fact, 4 percent to 12 percent of these first-degree relatives will test positive for celiac disease.

Gender Counts—How Food Allergies Discriminate

The battle of the sexes might rage for eternity, but when it comes to allergies, the lines are clearly drawn. With allergies of any kind, including food allergies, boys are more likely to develop a food allergy than girls. In one study from *Pediatric Allergy and Immunology,* researchers evaluated allergy-related disorders in two-year-old children and found that more boys than girls had an allergy-related disorder or positive allergy test.

By adulthood, however, the risk begins to favor women, as both asthma and allergies are more common in adult women than adult men. Nobody understands exactly why boys have a higher risk than girls or why adult women are more prone to allergies than adult men, but some theories suggest that sex hormones may play a role.

There is one exception to this rule: One type of delayed food allergy, eosinophilic esophagitis, which we'll discuss in chapter 6, consistently favors males over females across the age spectrum. In fact, 75 percent of the reported cases occur in white males, according to the North American Society for Pediatric Gastroenterology, Hepatology and Nutrition.

Health Conditions That Increase Your Risk of Food Intolerances

While food intolerances can—and often do—develop on their own, certain illnesses can raise your risk of developing a food intolerance. In fact, virtually any disease involving the small intestine can increase your risk of developing a food intolerance. This includes diseases like Crohn's disease, celiac disease, acute or chronic gastroenteritis, and autoimmune diseases.

Why do these diseases make you more vulnerable? Without getting too technical, all of these diseases cause inflammation of the small intestines, which leads to decreased brush-border digestive enzymes. The brush

Organ Transplant Recipients, Beware

Another group that appears to be at risk of developing a food allergy are children who have undergone solid organ transplants, specifically the liver or small bowel. Some studies have suggested this may be a result of the immunosuppressants used. It may also be caused by the specific organs that are transplanted. Why? Simply put, some organs are more involved in immune activity than others.

border provides enzymes that digest and absorb various food components. When that barrier system is compromised, your body doesn't produce as many enzymes. As a result, the food components that cause problems go undigested, leaving you more susceptible to developing a food intolerance.

chapter 3

Are Food Sensitivities
on the Rise?

When Bob Dylan released his hit single "The Times They Are A-Changin'" in 1964, he might as well have been writing about food sensitivities. That's because incidents of food sensitivities have undergone a huge change in the past few decades.

Think back to when you were a kid. Do you remember hearing anybody talk about food sensitivities or food allergies? Did you ever have a friend who was so allergic to peanuts you couldn't eat peanut butter and jelly sandwiches around him or her? Or did your mom avoid ice cream because she was lactose intolerant? Chances are, unless you're currently under the age of ten, probably not.

Yet you don't have to go back to your childhood to realize how different things were. Just ten, maybe even as little as five, years ago, you didn't hear as much about food sensitivities. Today, however, is a different story.

To some extent, food allergies have become a public health issue that affects all of us. Even if you don't have a food allergy, you might encounter the issue when flying on an airplane, sending your child to school, or going out to eat. In fact, if you thought about how many people you know who say they have a food intolerance or food allergy, you might be surprised to see how many people you can name.

Of course, all of this is welcome relief for people who do suffer from food sensitivities. Imagine for a minute if you're the mother of an eight-year-old boy who's allergic to peanuts. Wouldn't you have an easier time sending your son to school if you knew his environment was safe and wouldn't put him at risk for anaphylactic shock? The same could be said for an adult woman who has gluten intolerance. She no doubt appreciates that restaurants are catering to her sensitivity and that grocery stores now stock an entire section of gluten-free foods, since it means she has more options when she eats.

While increased awareness is good news for people with food sensitivities, it does beg some questions: Are food sensitivities on the upswing? Or are we just more aware of food sensitivities, leading more people to report them to doctors? Let's do a little number crunching to find out.

Why Food Intolerances May Not Be as Widespread as You Think

In an odd way, health conditions and their diagnosis are often subject to fads. These days, it's almost trendy to say you have a food intolerance.

Of course, there's no question that the number of people who think they have a food intolerance is high—and seemingly on the rise. Unfortunately, though, unlike food allergies, we can't tell you how many people suffer from food intolerances. Intolerances probably are more common than food allergies, but for several reasons, including the fact that most intolerances are impossible to definitively diagnose, firm numbers on how many people suffer don't exist. Yet we can draw some conclusions from our own patients.

In Dr. Qian's office, roughly 60 percent to 70 percent of the people who come to see him do so because they feel sick after eating and suspect they have a food intolerance. (Although as an allergist Dr. Wayne does see individuals with food intolerances, they're more likely to see Dr. Qian because he's a gastroenterologist.) And that number has certainly increased in recent years. Yet while some of these individuals do have food intolerances, the majority may not. So why do so many people think they have a food intolerance when, in reality, they do not? Let's look at some possible explanations.

For starters, what people think is a food intolerance often winds up being another health condition. In some cases, it could be a food allergy. More commonly, though, that person might be suffering from a health condition that has similar symptoms to a food intolerance. A classic example is irritable bowel syndrome (IBS), which affects about 20 percent of the adult population in the United States, according to the National Institute of Diabetes and Digestive and Kidney Diseases. Although researchers have yet to pinpoint exact causes of IBS, some believe that people with IBS have a sensitive colon that reacts to certain foods and stress. The immune system as well as the nervous system might also be involved.

Symptoms of IBS include abdominal pain, diarrhea, bloating, and a feeling of gas in the intestines. Surprisingly, these are the same symptoms you might experience if you have a food intolerance. To make matters more confusing, treatment of IBS often involves changing the diet. In fact, when people with IBS stop eating a certain food, they usually feel better, at least for a while. No wonder people with IBS often suspect they have a food intolerance! Yet the two are different. While people with food intolerances generally have reproducible reactions to foods, if you have IBS, your reactions to the same foods may vary depending on other factors, including emotional stress.

Stress, in fact, might be another condition that's causing your body to react to food differently. It's a fact, after all, that chronic stress can lead to problems in the gastrointestinal tract, including diarrhea and stomach pain. However, if you don't know this, stress won't hit your radar as a cause for your negative reaction to food, and so, once again, you might simply assume you have a food intolerance.

Health conditions aside, increased awareness of food intolerances could also be playing a role. After all, whether you're at the grocery store or a restaurant, it's becoming harder to go anywhere without hearing about food intolerances. That increased awareness, although beneficial for many individuals as we've already pointed out, may cause a heightened sense of alarm. Because people are more aware of food intolerances, they're more suspicious—and quicker to jump to conclusions—if they do experience an adverse reaction to food. It's easier to conclude that your negative reaction to a food is a food intolerance than to find other explanations, like food spoilage. Ironically, increased awareness of this medical issue may even be influencing the conclusions doctors are drawing.

Gluten intolerance is a prime example of increased awareness, as restaurants and grocery stores around the country have stepped up their efforts to meet consumer demands for gluten-free foods. The next time you go out to eat, notice if the restaurant offers gluten-free choices. In all likelihood, it probably does, as leading chains like Applebee's, P. F. Chang's, Ruby Tuesday, the Old Spaghetti Factory, and Olive Garden now offer gluten-free menus.

Or stroll through the grocery store, and keep your eyes peeled for the gluten-free section. It's tough to miss these days, especially since this section seems to be growing bigger by the second. In fact, between 2006 and 2010, the gluten-free food and beverage market grew 30 percent, reaching an estimated $2.6 billion in retail sales, and it's predicted that the growth will continue over the next five years.

That increased awareness may also be driving people to undergo blood tests and other tests to diagnose food intolerances. We'll discuss this more in chapter 4, when we take a closer look at food intolerances, but suffice it to say that there aren't any studies to show that these tests hold merit. These tests also aren't as accurate as people are often led to believe. As a result, mainstream medicine doesn't currently put much faith in these tests. Yet that hasn't stopped individuals who are concerned about their health (as they should be) from sometimes making big changes in their diet that can carry significant costs.

Finally, there is another possible cause for your woes with food: anxiety. We see many individuals who have had a bad reaction to food and begin to worry so much about the possibility of having an intolerance that they almost talk themselves into it. As a result, they experience negative symptoms whenever they eat. Of course, they could have an intolerance or even another unrelated medical condition, which is why you should always chat with your doctor to rule out definitive health conditions.

Bottom line is this: Outside a few intolerances that are well defined, we simply don't know much about the prevalence of food intolerances, largely because we don't have rigorous diagnostic criteria to define them. We know the number of perceived incidents is high, but, for the above reasons, they're almost certainly less than the self-reported numbers would suggest. Moreover, apart from celiac disease, there's no firm data to suggest they're increasing.

This is why keeping a food diary, as we mentioned in chapter 1, is so helpful. Before you start extensively limiting your diet, you want hard data to support that it's really worth the cost—financially, socially, and perhaps nutritionally—that comes with it.

What the Numbers Show About Food Allergies

When you start looking at food allergies, however, a somewhat clearer picture emerges. Food allergies aren't as common as food intolerances, but, unlike most food intolerances, we do have better numbers on how many people suffer from food allergies.

According to the Centers for Disease Control and Prevention, about 2 percent of American adults have a food allergy. Among children under eighteen years old, 3.9 percent are affected.

Those numbers, though, may need to be adjusted. A surprising new study from the journal *Pediatrics* estimates that as many as 8 percent of children under eighteen, or about one in thirteen American children, may have a food allergy. That means that at least twelve million of us, including three million children between the ages of five and seventeen (and more if the above study is correct), have a food allergy, and, as we'll soon reveal, the prevalence appears to be rising.

Even with food allergies, though, there's a discrepancy between how many people think they have food allergies and how many people have a diagnosed food allergy. In a study from the *Journal of Allergy and Clinical Immunology,* researchers found that as many as 35 percent of people surveyed indicated that they had a food allergy. These were self-reported food allergies, meaning that an actual diagnosis wasn't confirmed. This is roughly five to ten times the actual rates we cited above.

So why is there such a difference between actual statistics and self-reported numbers of food allergy sufferers? Again, we can blame several culprits.

First and foremost, the definition of food allergy itself is largely misunderstood and frequently misused. For instance, how many times have you heard people joke that they're "allergic" to work or even another person? Of course, they're not really allergic to work per se (although technically they could be allergic to something in their work environment) or to a person, but because it's easy to toss the word around, the true meaning of allergy has gotten muddled.

Plus, people are likely to call any adverse reaction to a food a food allergy, even though it could be a food intolerance or something unrelated to either a food allergy or a food intolerance. Lactose intolerance is a good example, since people often confuse lactose intolerance with milk allergy.

The medical community has also contributed to the problem. In some settings, individuals are given food allergy tests that lack the accuracy or validation of other tests, like the food challenge we often do in our office. (We'll discuss this in more detail in chapter 7, but in a food challenge, we ask you to consume the food we suspect is triggering your allergies.) Results from these tests often suggest that the patient may have a food allergy.

However, without having done a food challenge (which should be done, by the way, only in controlled settings and with medical help nearby), a food allergy often can't be confirmed. In fact, the general consensus in the medical community is that there's an overestimation of food allergies.

In a *Journal of the American Medical Association* study, researchers found that people who had positive skin-prick or blood tests actually had less than a 50 percent chance of having that allergy. This means that having a positive allergy test isn't the same as having an allergy, and this misunderstanding leads many doctors to over-diagnose their patients.

To explain, allergy tests screen for immunoglobin E (IgE) antibodies, which are produced by the immune system and can cause allergic reactions. While it's true that IgE antibodies have to be present for immediate allergic reactions to occur, their presence may be irrelevant if a person has no physical reaction to the suspected allergen. In other words, the presence of IgE is necessary but not sufficient alone for most forms of allergic reactions. That's why although the tests may accurately identify the presence of IgE to a food allergen, they may still be falsely positive from a clinical perspective.

Even the gold-standard test of food challenges has limitations, since symptoms consistent with allergic reactions like hives or shortness of breath may in some rare cases be caused by anxiety. Consider, for instance, this study from the journal *Allergy,* in which researchers conducted a double-blind, placebo-controlled food challenge where children were exposed to a substance they were likely to be allergic to. None of the 105 children in the study, however, knew whether they were exposed to the real allergen or the placebo.

In the end, seventeen children experienced symptoms in response to the placebo, meaning that they developed falsely positive reactions after being exposed to the placebo, which shouldn't have caused any reaction. Could anxiety have contributed? It seems likely.

So Why Am I Hearing More About Peanut (and Other Food) Allergies These Days?

It's not a figment of your imagination: Food allergies are indeed on the rise. According to the Centers for Disease Control and Prevention, the number of children with food allergies between 1997 and 2007 increased by 18 percent. While 2.3 million children under the age of eighteen were reported to have a food or digestive allergy in 1997, that number rose to approximately three million children just a decade later.

Researchers don't have firm answers, and theories about what may be fueling this rise in food allergies are difficult to test, but here are some of the leading ideas:

Theory #1: The Hygiene Hypothesis

Cleanliness may be next to godliness, but Americans have taken their infatuation with being clean to a new level. Just look at all the antibacterial products on the market. There's even antibacterial toothpaste, of all things! We've essentially launched a war against germs. Unfortunately, though, our obsession with dirt could be making us sick, which is the basis of a theory called the hygiene hypothesis, now the most widely accepted explanation for why allergies are on the rise.

Simply put, the hygiene hypothesis suggests that we're not exposing our immune systems to enough dirt and germs. Because we live in such tidy environments, we're exposed to fewer bugs, and the less our immune systems have to worry about fending off germs and bacteria—which is, after all, one of their main functions— the less tolerant they may be of ordinarily harmless items like allergens.

Take, for instance, having pets in the house. Studies have shown that the presence of pets in the house is protective against allergies in general. The reason? Pets may increase your exposure to numerous germs, and because your immune system is busy fending off those germs, it doesn't react to other allergens it's encountering.

Similar findings come from studies of the effect of birth order. Firstborns are actually at higher risk of allergies overall, perhaps because younger siblings benefit from increased exposure to germs that have been introduced by the older sibling.

So does this mean you should roll around in the dirt more, even clean your house less? Not necessarily. As popular as this theory is, it does have its limitations, including the fact that the evidence supporting it comes from observations, not from actual studies, which suggests that factors other than a clean environment may be triggering allergies.

Theory #2: Changes in Food Manufacturing

Some experts speculate that changes in the way food, particularly peanuts, is processed may be inflating the number of people who suffer from food allergies. For example, the prevalence of peanut allergy in China is much lower than that of the United States, even though the Chinese eat just as many peanuts per capita as Americans do.

One explanation: In the United States, peanuts are often roasted, whereas in China, peanuts are commonly boiled. Some studies with animals have suggested that roasting peanuts may alter the protein in peanuts enough to trigger allergic reactions more effectively which might explain why peanut allergies are less common in China.

There's also speculation that changes in the way peanut butter is made could be fueling the rise in allergies, but, to date, there haven't been any good studies to prove this theory.

Theory #3: Insufficient Amounts of Nutrients

It's no secret that Americans aren't the healthiest of eaters, and while those unhealthy eating habits are undoubtedly contributing to the obesity epidemic and related medical conditions, the lack of certain nutrients in the American diet may be fueling allergies, too. Three nutrients have attracted the most interest when it comes to increasing allergies: vitamin D, vitamin A, and folate. Of those three nutrients, vitamin D has been the most widely studied.

Vitamin D is a hot topic these days. If you've watched TV or read a magazine in recent months, you've probably caught some of the hoopla surrounding vitamin D, which helps build strong bones and regulate the immune system. While sunlight is the most significant source of vitamin D, you can also get it from food—salmon, mackerel, and milk (because of vitamin D fortification) are great sources—and a vitamin D supplement.

Recent studies have suggested that low levels of vitamin D may be linked to cardiovascular disease, diabetes, obesity, autoimmune disorders, even increased incidents of cold and flu. Furthermore, medical researchers increasingly believe that a large percentage of the population, particularly in temperate latitudes, is deficient in vitamin D and that levels fluctuate with the seasons. It should be little wonder, then, that we're looking at vitamin D in relation to food allergies. So what's the connection? Once again, let's look at what current studies have found.

In one study, researchers at Harvard found that EpiPen prescriptions were more common in cities in the United States at higher latitudes and with lower UVB exposures than more southern cities, which may suggest a link between vitamin D levels and allergies. Bakersfield, California, which records 273 days of sunshine annually, had the lowest number of EpiPen prescriptions, while Bellingham, Washington, which averages only 71 sunny days a year, had the highest number of EpiPen prescriptions.

While this data is certainly intriguing, it's not enough for us to recommend vitamin D supplementation based on food allergy alone. Nor do we recommend screening for vitamin D deficiency just because a child has a food allergy. Although there are reasons to screen for vitamin D deficiencies in some food-allergic children— for instance, if they're not consuming milk because of an allergy—their food allergy alone isn't enough to warrant screening.

Vitamin D isn't the only nutrient that's being implicated in allergies. Two other nutrients that may play a role in allergies are vitamin A and folic acid: too much of the former and not enough of the latter.

Vitamin A (found in fat-free milk, cheese pizza, cooked chicken, beef, and eggs) can potentially enhance the kind of immune response needed to cause allergies, although this hasn't been directly linked to food allergy. Meanwhile, folates (found in fortified breakfast cereals, great northern beans, asparagus, raw spinach, wheat germ, and canned tomato juice) are important because low levels of them have been associated with increased allergies.

Theory #4: Food Introduction

Over the last decade, food introduction, the age at which children are introduced to allergy-prone foods, has undergone quite a bit of controversy, especially considering its role in the development of food allergies. Until recently, we advised parents to delay the introduction of the most commonly allergenic foods, like egg, milk, wheat, peanut, soy, fish, and shellfish. The rationale was partly based on ideas about the immunity of the gut and immune systems of young children. Small but influential studies also suggested that delaying the introduction of these foods was potentially protective against food allergies and related problems like eczema. Yet more— and better—research is beginning to reveal that late introduction of some of these foods may actually be increasing, or at the very least not lowering, the prevalence of food allergies.

In a widely cited study of ten thousand Jewish children, researchers compared the rate of peanut allergies in children in London with peanut allergy rates among children in Tel Aviv. The results, which appeared in the *Journal of Allergy and Clinical Immunology*, showed that the Jewish children in the greater London area were almost ten times as likely to have a peanut allergy as their counterparts in Tel Aviv.

Why such a difference between the two groups of children? Even though the children shared similar genetic backgrounds and allergies, including food allergies, which are comparable in Israel and the United Kingdom, children in Israel are generally introduced to peanuts at a younger age than children in the United Kingdom. There's a popular peanut-containing snack food in Israel called Bamba that kids start eating when they're infants. Researchers concluded that this early exposure may make kids less sensitive to peanuts, which could decrease their risk of developing a food allergy.

Yet another significant study examined milk allergy in children. Researchers from Tel Aviv University tracked the feeding history of over thirteen thousand infants. The results were telling: Women who introduced cow's milk to their infants in the first fifteen days of life almost entirely eliminated incidence of allergy to cow milk protein in their babies.

Similarly, another study found that infants who weren't introduced to eggs until they were ten months or older had a higher risk of developing a food allergy than infants who were introduced to eggs between four and six months. This is the theme of a number of recent studies: When a relation is found between food introduction and the development of food allergy, earlier introduction is associated with lower, not higher, rates of food allergy.

As a result of all this research, food introduction guidelines have shifted. The American Academy of Pediatrics, which a little less than a decade ago endorsed delayed introduction of eggs, peanuts, tree nuts, and fish, no longer believes that there's enough convincing evidence that delaying the introduction of certain foods has a protective benefit. Currently, it recommends introducing solid foods to infants between the ages of four and six months, regardless of family history of food allergy or other risk factors.

part II

Food Intolerances

chapter 4

Food Intolerances 101

We don't need to tell you that having a food intolerance is frustrating. Perhaps you've already experienced a lot of aggravation in your search for answers. Yet the problem—and we hate to keep bringing this up—is that we, as doctors and allergy specialists, simply don't know that much about many food intolerances.

With a few exceptions, we can't tell you what causes them. We can't tell you why you developed this intolerance. For most food intolerances, we can't even tell you with real certainty that you truly have a food intolerance. Often, the most helpful thing we can do is rule out some of the worst things and then tell you what we suspect you might have. How's that for advanced medical science?

Add to this all the erroneous misinformation floating around out there about food intolerances, and it can really boggle your mind. As soon as you think you have one thing figured out, you hear something that contradicts what you thought you knew, and the wild-goose chase begins again.

We can't promise you'll never go on that chase again, but we'll try to make your struggles easier as we bring some clarity to your issues. In this chapter, we'll discuss the symptoms we believe are most consistent with food intolerances, how you can figure out which foods might be bothering you, and what diagnostic tests might do you the most good along with tests you'll want to avoid.

Why We Know So Little About Food Intolerances

Although food allergies are well studied, research on most food intolerances is practically nonexistent. It's not that we don't want to know what's going on with food intolerances. We wish we could unlock the mystery of food intolerances, and, we hope someday we will. It's just that there are numerous obstacles in the way.

For starters, nobody understands the mechanisms behind most food intolerances. While we know that certain intolerances like lactose, fructose, and sucrose may be caused by a lack of digestive enzymes or an inability to absorb some sugars, we don't know much, if anything, about the causes behind many other intolerances. Without these clues and firm diagnostic criteria, researchers have few starting points and little incentive to launch studies.

Plus, given the broad definition of food intolerance, knowing what to include in any study would be nearly impossible. We can only summarize the experiences of our patients and apply what we currently understand about human physiology.

Identifying Possible Suspects

Although we don't know what causes many food intolerances, we're not completely in the dark, especially when it comes to intolerances to lactose, sucrose, and alcohol. People who have these intolerances are missing a certain digestive enzyme, and the lack of that enzyme causes you to physically feel bad.

In a normal functioning digestive system, food is broken down into small pieces with the help of enzymes in your saliva, stomach, and digestive tract. Your body then goes to work absorbing the food, taking out the nutrients it needs to maintain itself. For instance, when you drink milk, an enzyme called lactase breaks down a sugar in milk called lactose into simpler forms that are then absorbed into the bloodstream.

Yet people with intolerances to lactose and sucrose lack the enzyme that will properly break down these two sugars, which is why it's impossible to outgrow these intolerances. As a result, these sugars, which should have been digested and absorbed by the body, sit in the gut, where they ferment and generate gasses that cause bloating, cramping, diarrhea, and nausea.

In the case of alcohol-intolerant individuals, the same chain of events happens. Because these individuals lack the proper enzymes to metabolize the toxins in alcohol, they suffer symptoms, although they're slightly different from the ones that lactose- and sucrose-intolerant individuals experience. With alcohol intolerance, common symptoms include nasal congestion, flushed face, and rapid heartbeat.

How Do You Know If You Have a Food Intolerance?

That's, of course, the million-dollar question, which is why we should revisit our definition of food intolerance: a reproducible, adverse reaction to a food that's not the direct result of an immune response. Let's break that down a little more.

First and foremost, you need to have some adverse reaction to food, and it needs to be reproducible. In other words, after you've had a negative reaction to a food, you should have a bad reaction when you eat that food again. Symptoms don't have to be the same or as severe each time, but you should have some type of reaction. Those symptoms will most likely include some of the following:

- Nausea
- Stomach pain
- Gas, cramps, or bloating
- Vomiting
- Diarrhea
- Heartburn
- Headache
- Migraine

You then need to figure out if the immune system is involved to rule out food allergy, which is a bit tricky and requires testing by an allergist or gastroenterologist. If all the tests come back negative (as Kathy's did in chapter 1), that speaks against a food allergy. It would then be logical to conclude that you have a food intolerance. (Of course, the caveat here is that a positive test may still not actually prove that you have an allergy.)

You may also go through some simple trial and

error to better understand the problem. We should note, though, that certain warning signs warrant immediate medical help, since these can indicate much more serious problems.

If you have a family history of celiac disease, experience symptoms of immediate food allergy (like itchiness, hives, respiratory distress, coughing, sudden onset of vomiting, diarrhea, or abdominal pain within a couple of hours after eating certain foods) or have symptoms that may be related to a delayed food allergy (like difficulty swallowing, food becoming stuck when swallowing, chronic chest pain, heartburn, vomiting, diarrhea, constipation, weight loss, or abdominal pain), you need to see your doctor. You might also consult with an allergist or gastroenterologist.

These symptoms may be caused by conditions that need to be treated by a medical expert. In some cases, going untreated could put you at risk for serious health consequences. Other warning signs that might indicate potentially serious diseases include weight loss, anemia, chronic fatigue, bloody stools, chronic fevers, and night sweats.

If, though, you don't have any of these serious symptoms and think you've figured out what foods are bothering you, consider a trial elimination diet for one to three months, where you completely avoid the suspicious food or foods. If your symptoms disappear, you may have identified the culprit correctly, and you should continue avoiding that food. Again, if you don't have any of the more serious symptoms we've discussed above, you may want to confirm the culprit by a trial reintroduction of that food.

Just maintain a healthy dose of skepticism. Some symptoms like gastrointestinal upset or migraines are common and come and go for reasons we can't identify. Try not to jump to conclusions, and if you start manipulating your diet extensively, consider consulting with a registered dietitian to make sure you're meeting your nutritional needs. (To find a dietitian in your area, visit the Academy of Nutrition and Dietetics at www .eatright.org.)

But what if your symptoms return or you don't know what foods are bothering you in the first place? Start a food diary, which we discussed in chapter 1, so you can start narrowing down what foods might be a problem. To review, write down everything you eat and drink every day for several weeks, including how much you consume and any symptoms you experience. Review your food diary after a few weeks, and you may be able to spot the foods that are bothering you.

Bear in mind, though, that the culprit is often a single ingredient you need to identify before you can see a pattern. For instance, some people are sensitive to monosodium glutamate or caffeine. Yet if they don't know that those ingredients are present in various foods, they may not suspect those two food items.

To combat this, focus on symptoms like gastrointestinal changes that are most likely to be related to foods. Note how quickly after eating these symptoms begin, what the exact symptoms are, and how long it takes the symptoms to resolve. Symptoms that occur a long time after you've eaten a particular food are less likely to be directly related to that food.

With the exception of celiac disease or an intolerance called lactase deficiency, both of which are lifelong conditions, some less-defined food intolerances seem to resolve after several months. If you've been on an elimination diet, the only way you'll know if your intolerance has been resolved is by reintroducing a small amount of your trigger food back into your diet. Ironically, this usually isn't a planned event for most people. One day, they accidentally eat a food they previously couldn't tolerate, and because they don't have a reaction, they begin eating that food more regularly again.

If you don't want to wait until this happens, and in the absence of those warning signs we discussed above, you may consider introducing the food back into your diet slowly, eating only a small amount of the food at a time. If you're avoiding multiple foods, don't introduce several foods at once. Otherwise, if symptoms recur, you could be confused about which food caused the reaction.

If you don't have any reactions, you can gradually increase how much you eat of that food. However, if you do have a reaction and feel sick, go back to the elimination diet. Then wait several months before testing your body again to see if it's lost its sensitivity.

Can a Food Intolerance Be Diagnosed?

Look online for the answer to this question, and you'll probably find dozens of tests that promise to diagnose your food intolerance. Unfortunately, they're all completely unvalidated.

For starters, there's the hair test, where your hair is tested for mineral deficiencies, which is supposed to tell you what food intolerances you have, and muscle kinesiology, which measures your muscle's response to potentially offensive foods. Two other tests are the live blood microscopic analysis and energy mapping, but to be honest, we have little understanding about what these tests are designed to do. As we've already noted, although these tests are offered by various individuals, most of them have little scientific validation. This is also true for another test called the mediator release test (MRT). You may have heard more about this test, as it's becoming increasingly popular. Because numerous nutritionists and some physicians are promoting it (and many of our patients ask us about it), we'll spend a little more time discussing it.

Essentially, this test measures your body's production of a type of antibody called immunoglobin G (IgG) to 150 different foods and chemicals. If the test reveals that you have a high IgG response to one or several foods, the claim is that you have an intolerance to those foods.

Yet here's the problem with this test: While IgG helps your body defend against infection, it also registers exposures to food proteins, so that for every food you eat, your body produces IgG to that food. Roughly speaking, the more you eat a certain food, the higher your IgG level to that food will be, and, conversely, the less you eat a food, the lower your IgG level to that food will be. Although your body views all foods as invaders (which they are, since you have to introduce them to the body), the IgG your body makes in response to food hasn't been shown to cause any problems.

Imagine, for instance, that you're a meat eater, and

you've just consumed a steak dinner. If meat is a staple in your diet, you'll probably have a high IgG response to beef. However, if you were to measure IgG levels for beef in a vegetarian who hasn't consumed meat in decades, if at all, IgG levels to beef in that individual would be practically nonexistent.

Even though IgG is elevated with exposure to food, no peer-reviewed data that we're aware of demonstrates that elevated IgG levels cause or are consistently associated with any food intolerance, which is why the medical community hasn't embraced the MRT test. There may come a day when research reveals that IgG does play some role in specific food intolerances (in which case they would be reclassified as a type of food allergy), but right now that data doesn't exist.

Still, some of our patients have chosen to undergo the MRT test. There's no harm to your health in getting it done, but it could damage your wallet, since the test costs several hundred dollars and isn't covered by insurance. Furthermore, if you're advised to restrict your diet, that's not a trivial thing. Dietary restrictions are time consuming, expensive, socially isolating, and could have a negative impact on your nutrition.

Although these tests may sound enticing, they haven't been subjected to controlled testing and, as a result, are unproven. And because they're not consistent with what we currently understand about human physiology, we don't advise spending your money on them.

The Hydrogen Breath Test for Lactose, Fructose, and Sucrose Intolerances

Fortunately, though, the news isn't all negative when it comes to diagnosing food intolerances, for there are tests that offer some accuracy.

One of the standards is the hydrogen breath test, which is used for diagnosing lactose, fructose, and sucrose intolerances. In people who have these intolerances, lactose, fructose, and sucrose move into the intestines where they sit and ferment. That fermentation creates gasses—hydrogen and methane—that pass into the bloodstream and eventually reach the lungs. Through the hydrogen breath test, we can measure these gasses to determine if you have an intolerance.

Here's how the test works: If your doctor suspects you have one of these intolerances, you'll fast overnight. In the morning, you'll return to the doctor's office to blow air into a bag, which will measure your baseline hydrogen and methane levels. After this initial blow, you'll consume a drink with either lactose, fructose, or sucrose, depending on which is suspected to be causing your problems—for instance, you'll drink about as much lactose as there is in a gallon of milk!—and then every thirty minutes for three hours, you'll blow air into the bag.

During the test, you'll also answer questions about how you're feeling. For instance, do you have any bloating? nausea? abdominal symptoms? In the end, if hydrogen and methane levels are elevated in your body and you've experienced symptoms during the test, then there's a good chance you have one of these intolerances.

Note, though, that 1 percent of the population doesn't have hydrogen-producing bacteria in the gut. Even though their hydrogen levels will be normal, these individuals will still have discomfort during the breath test (i.e., nausea, bloating, abdominal pain, diarrhea, and flatulence), which is enough to conclude that they have an intolerance.

There's also the possibility that your test results could be negative, even though you're still having symptoms. For instance, 30 percent to 40 percent of people with clinical symptoms of lactose intolerance will have a negative breath test. For these individuals, we don't know what's causing their woes, although we can pretty much rule out lactose intolerance.

To diagnose lactose and sucrose intolerance in

infants and children under five years old, we use the stool-acidity test. When undigested lactose remains in the digestive tract, it creates acids that are present in a stool sample. Glucose, often the result of unabsorbed lactose and sucrose, might also be present in the sample. While this can't tell us whether the child is suffering from lactose or sucrose intolerance, the test does offer some clues about what might be causing any digestive problems.

Diagnosing Celiac Disease

Tests are also available for people whom we suspect have celiac disease. The first test is a blood test in which we measure antibody levels—we're looking at two specifically, one called tissue transglutaminase (TTG), and another called anti-endyomysial antibodies (EMA)—to see if any are elevated. To keep this test as accurate as possible, you'll be asked to continue eating your normal diet, including any foods that contain gluten, for at least four weeks. Otherwise, if you eliminate gluten, your antibody levels could be normal, which will delay your diagnosis.

If the blood test confirms that you do have high antibody levels—a whopping 90 percent of people with untreated celiac disease have elevated antibody levels,

The Many Faces of Food Intolerances

So that you can get a better sense of how a food intolerance is diagnosed and managed, meet two food-intolerant individuals.

Case study #1: Jack

Jack is a forty-seven-year-old who's had trouble with abdominal discomfort, bloating, and diarrhea for several years. His symptoms, which usually occur a couple of hours after eating, seem to get worse after he consumes any food containing dairy, including milk, cheese, yogurt, or ice cream. Yet after a few bouts of diarrhea and passing lots of gas, he feels much better.

His primary care physician recommended a lactose breath test, which has shown that Jack has lactose intolerance. As a result, he no longer drinks regular milk, instead consuming lactose-free milk, and he takes lactase pills whenever he eats dairy. He's now symptom-free.

Case study #2: Amy

At forty-two, Amy felt bloated all the time, especially after eating. She also had abdominal pain, occasional nausea,

(continued)

and alternating bouts of constipation and diarrhea. Yet she was always careful about what she ate, following a healthy diet with lots of fruits, vegetables, and water. She also exercised at least three times a week.

Her primary care physician ran blood tests on her, which were normal. She then underwent an abdominal X-ray, and because it showed some constipation, she was sent to a gastroenterologist, who ran additional tests. Yet an upper endoscopy and colonoscopy were normal. However, a hydrogen breath test revealed a possible fructose intolerance. She was also diagnosed with irritable bowel syndrome (IBS).

Since then, she's tweaked her diet by avoiding foods and drinks with fructose, especially in the form of corn syrup, and giving up chewing gum. (An ingredient in gum called sorbitol could make her feel bad.) She also takes a stool softener to manage the IBS and now feels much better. She's having regular bowel movements and rarely complains about abdominal discomfort.

which are rarely elevated in people who don't have celiac disease—your doctor will send you to a gastroenterologist to have a small-intestine biopsy, collected during an upper endoscopy. The test involves swallowing a small,

> ## Tips for Steering Clear of Food Intolerance Reactions
>
> - Learn which foods are causing your problems; then experiment to see how much, if any, of that food your body can handle.
> - Read food labels and check ingredient lists for your trigger foods.
> - When dining out, always ask your server or host how foods have been prepared. Descriptions on menus often aren't detailed enough to give you the full picture.

flexible instrument with a camera, which the gastroenterologist uses to check for damage to the villi.

Villi are fingerlike structures in the lining of the small intestine. They allow the small intestine to absorb nutrients. In people with celiac disease, these villi become flattened, rendering them unable to absorb those nutrients. After you eliminate gluten from your diet, though, the villi resume their normal growth pattern, and your body can properly absorb nutrients.

chapter 5

Getting a Handle on Common Intolerances

You might say that food intolerances are politically correct: They honestly don't discriminate. Not only can anybody develop a food intolerance but also anybody can develop an intolerance to a wide variety of foods.

While that certainly doesn't make things easier if you're trying to figure out which foods are causing you trouble, the most likely culprits tend to be commonly eaten foods. That's why gluten and lactose are probably two of the top troublemakers in the United States. Head to another country, however, and you would no doubt find that the most common intolerances are different, which suggests that as eating habits shift, so, too, do food intolerances.

We're not saying, though, that you can prevent food

intolerances simply by avoiding eating too much of one food. At this point, we don't know enough about food intolerances to say whether any of them can be prevented. Yet we can tell you how to manage them. Let's take a look at nine of the most common intolerances.

Got Milk? You Could Have Lactose Intolerance

If you suffer from lactose intolerance, you're not alone. Estimates indicate that anywhere from thirty to fifty million Americans are lactose intolerant, and, as we discussed in chapter 2, certain populations have higher incidents of lactose intolerance, including Asians, African Americans, and Hispanics. These individuals lack an enzyme called lactase to properly digest lactose, a sugar in milk and milk products. That lactose remains undigested in the gut, where hungry bacteria feed on it, fermenting it, and generating gas that causes physical discomfort. The most common symptoms are abdominal pain, diarrhea, flatulence, and bloating.

Of course, many people confuse lactose intolerance with milk allergy. The two, however, are different. With milk allergy, the immune system has developed a sensitivity to milk protein, which then triggers allergic reactions. Yet with lactose intolerance, the immune system isn't involved, because the lack of this digestive enzyme is the sole cause.

Yet here's the interesting thing about lactose intolerance: In general, everybody's born with the lactase enzyme and can usually tolerate lactose, which is a good thing since milk provides crucial nutrients for babies. Yet for people who develop lactose intolerance, that enzyme begins to diminish as they age, which may explain why lactose intolerance often doesn't occur until adulthood. By the time these individuals are fourteen or fifteen years old, that enzyme has diminished by almost half. At that point, their bodies begin reacting, and they can no longer tolerate foods they used to eat.

Although this enzyme continues to diminish with age, it's never eliminated completely. Yet how much of the enzyme remains varies from one person to another. That's why many individuals with lactose intolerance don't have to give up lactose entirely. They just have to cut back and learn how much they can tolerate. For some people, that might mean eating one scoop of ice cream without any woes while others might not be able to eat one bite of a grilled cheese sandwich without feeling sick. If you suspect you have lactose intolerance, don't rely on self-diagnosis. After all, if you don't have lactose intolerance but mistakenly cut all dairy products from your diet, you could be unnecessarily depriving your body of nutrients, including calcium, vitamins A and D, riboflavin, and phosphorus. As a result, you could set yourself up for health problems like osteoporosis down the road. Instead, ask your physician about getting tested.

Once you have a diagnosis, you can control your symptoms through dietary changes. Although small children who are born with a lactase deficiency shouldn't eat any foods containing lactose, most older children and adults don't have to avoid lactose completely.

Yet you'll have to experiment to determine exactly how much lactose you can tolerate. Many lactose-intolerant individuals can consume up to a cup of milk with minimal side effects, especially when consumed with food. Larger amounts can often be consumed if you spread them out throughout the day and drink them with food. Know, too, that dairy products like low-fat or fat-free hard cheese, cottage cheese, ice cream, and yogurt often contain less lactose than milk and may cause fewer symptoms.

You can also buy lactose-free and lactose-reduced milk and milk products at most grocery stores. In these products, the lactase enzyme has been added, which either eliminates or reduces lactose.

Another option? Pop an over-the-counter lactase supplement as you eat. The supplement will help you digest any lactose you're eating. If you forget to take it as you eat, you can still take it after eating, which could help ease any symptoms that have developed. Try to take it within thirty minutes of eating, although you might be okay taking it even an hour later, especially if you have slower digestive function.

Then learn to spot hidden lactose in foods, especially if you have a low tolerance to lactose. Any food containing milk, nonfat milk solids, skim milk, butter, cream, lactose, or whey should be avoided. Other terms that could indicate lactose include "milk by-products" and "nonfat dry milk powder."

Want help knowing what to eat and avoid? Follow this chart:

Food group:	Foods to eat:	Foods to avoid:
Milk	Soy milk; rice milk; oat milk; Lactaid 100 milk; soy cheese and Lactaid cheese; soy yogurt; yogurt, sour cream, cheese, or buttermilk if some lactose can be tolerated.	All milk and milk drinks, including whole, skim, low-fat, dried, evaporated, and condensed. Any type of yogurt, sour cream, frappés, shakes, and ice cream. All cheese and cheese dishes. (continued)

Food group:	Foods to eat:	Foods to avoid:
Beverages	Powdered, fruit-flavored drinks; tonics; sodas; juices; water.	Any beverages made with milk, eggnog, and hot chocolate.
Eggs	As desired. Do not prepare with butter or margarine that contains milk products.	Any eggs made with milk or butter or margarine that contains milk products.
Meat, poultry, fish	Any baked, broiled, roasted, boiled meat, poultry, or fish.	Creamed or breaded meat, fish, or poultry. Prepared meats may contain dried milk solids, including bologna, cold cuts, frankfurters, salami, commercially prepared fish sticks, and some sausage.

Food group:	Foods to eat:	Foods to avoid:
Breads	Breads made without milk, such as French bread, Italian bread, bagels, or pareve bread.	Any baked products made with milk such as muffins, biscuits, waffles, donuts, pancakes, sweet rolls, and loaf breads.
Cereal	Any made without milk. Pasta and rice prepared without milk.	Any prepared cereal that contains dry milk solids.
Vegetables	All cooked, canned, frozen, or fresh.	Any vegetable prepared with milk, butter, or margarine containing milk products, milk solids, bread, or bread crumbs. Cheese or cheese sauce.

(continued)

Food group:	Foods to eat:	Foods to avoid:
Fruits	All	None
Desserts	Any made without milk or milk products. Gelatin, fruit crisps, fruit-and-water ice sorbet, pie with fruit filling, angel food cake, Tofutti or soy ice cream, and rice ice cream.	All commercial cake and cookie mixes, ice cream, custard, puddings, ice milk or sherbets that contain milk. Frosting made with milk or butter, dessert sauces, cheesecake.
Soup	Any homemade or canned soup prepared without milk or milk products.	All creamed soups and chowders, cheese soup.
Fats	Milk-free margarine or pareve margarine, oils, nuts, peanut butter.	Butter or margarine containing milk products, some commercial salad dressings.

Food group:	Foods to eat:	Foods to avoid:
Seasonings	Sugar, honey, molasses, maple syrup, corn syrup, jelly, jam, hard candy, gumdrops, marshmallow, and mints. Salt, pepper, herbs, vinegar, catsup, relish, pickles, olives, coconut, and wheat germ. Artificial flavorings or extracts.	None

One other surprising place you'll find lactose? Medications. Lactose has been added to over 20 percent of prescription drugs and roughly 6 percent of over-the-counter medicines, according to the American Gastroenterological Association: Birth control pills and tablets for stomach acid and gas are two of the common offenders. If you suspect you are lactose intolerant, always ask your pharmacist about lactose in any medications you're taking.

As you're working to solve your lactose woes, you should also make sure your diet doesn't fall flat in calcium, which your body needs to grow and repair bones. Here's how much calcium you need:

Age	Calcium (milligrams/day)
0 to 6 months	200
7 to 12 months	260
1 to 3 years	700
4 to 8 years	1,000
9 to 18 years	1,300
19 to 50 years	1,000
51 to 70 years	1,000 men / 1,200 women
71+ years	1,200

Milk and other dairy products are the best sources of calcium. Yet if you've eliminated these foods from your diet, nondairy sources of calcium include canned sardines in oil (324 milligrams in three ounces), fortified orange juice (378 milligrams in six ounces), and cooked spinach (123 milligrams in one half cup). You can also take a calcium supplement, but talk with your doctor about this option.

The other concern? Vitamin D. Calcium, after all, is best absorbed and used in the body when enough vitamin D is present. However, if you've cut milk products, which are fortified with vitamin D, it's possible you may not be getting enough. How much do you need? Check out these recently updated recommendations from the Institute of Medicine:

Age (years)	Vitamin D (International Units/day)
1 to 3	600
4 to 8	600
9 to 18	600
19 to 50	600
51 to 71	600
71+	800

Although a cup of vitamin-D-fortified nonfat or reduced-fat milk contains roughly 100 IU, nondairy food sources of vitamin D include cooked sockeye salmon (447 IU in three ounces), cooked mackerel (388 IU in three ounces), canned tuna in water (154 IU in three ounces), vitamin-D-fortified orange juice (100 IU in one cup), and eggs (41 IU in one large egg). You can also take vitamin D supplements, but check with your doctor first.

When Sugar Isn't Sweet— Fructose Intolerance

Fructose is a sugar that occurs naturally in numerous foods, especially fruits, some vegetables, and honey. It's also found in table sugar and is used to sweeten many processed foods and beverages, including fruit juices and soft drinks.

Fructose intolerance, also called fructose malabsorption, is caused by lack of a digestive enzyme. People with irritable bowel syndrome are also prone to developing fructose intolerance, although whether they're deficient in the digestive enzyme isn't clear. When undigested fructose reaches the intestines, it reacts with naturally occurring bacteria and generates hydrogen gasses, causing diarrhea, gas, bloating, abdominal pain, and heartburn. Those gasses are then measured in the hydrogen breath test, which doctors use to determine if you have fructose intolerance.

To prevent these symptoms, avoid consuming fructose. That may not be as easy as it sounds, since fructose is found in numerous foods, including fruits, fruit juices, table sugar, sodas, and processed foods and drinks with high-fructose corn syrup.

Fortunately, though, many people can tolerate small amounts of fructose without any trouble. You'll have to experiment to determine how much your body can handle, but know that the small intestine has a limited capacity to absorb fructose, with about half of the population unable to absorb 25 grams. For instance, keeping in mind that 1,000 milligrams equals 1 gram, a cup of Kellogg's Raisin Bran contains 9,584 milligrams of fructose, while an ounce of a highly caffeinated soda could contain almost 30,000 milligrams.

Then, limit these foods in your diet: honey, processed foods, sodas and other drinks containing high-fructose corn syrup, foods that contain high-fructose corn syrup, and fruits and fruit juices.

Yet don't think you have to go cold turkey on all fruits and fruit juices. Because they have varying amounts of fructose, you can include some gut-friendly ones in your diet. They include strawberries, raspberries, blackberries, pineapple, kiwifruit, lemons, limes, rhubarbs, oranges, blueberries, avocados, grapes, honeydew melons, papayas, mandarin oranges, and tangelos. Meanwhile, those with the highest levels of fructose, which aren't as gut-friendly, include prunes, pears, cherries, peaches, apples, plums, grapes, dates, mangoes, watermelons, as well as apple and pear juice and apple cider.

One other note: Sorbitol is often used as an artificial sweetener in many food products, including chewing gum. Yet because sorbitol is converted to fructose during digestion, you should avoid it. However, other artificial sweeteners may be okay for you to use.

There's also another condition associated with fructose that's called fructosemia, or hereditary fructose intolerance. This is caused by another enzyme defect, and for infants it can be deadly. Without this enzyme, complicated chemical changes occur in the body, causing blood sugar to drop and dangerous substances to build up in the liver. Symptoms can include convulsions, excessive sleepiness, irritability, jaundice, poor feeding as a baby, problems after eating fruits and foods that contain fructose or sucrose, and vomiting. This is a severe illness that can lead to liver failure and, in some cases, death.

This isn't always the case, though. Dr. Qian once treated a four-year-old boy who refused to eat anything sweet, even vegetables. Other doctors had told his parents he was just being picky. His parents, however, weren't convinced and sought help from Dr. Qian, who did an endoscopy, which didn't reveal anything out of the ordinary. Yet when tested for the enzyme defect, the boy was found to be deficient. In the future, as long as he doesn't eat fructose, he'll suffer no ill consequences.

How this little boy survived infancy, though, is a miracle, which again underscores how mysterious these conditions can be.

Meet Sucrose Intolerance, a Close Cousin of Fructose Intolerance

Sucrose is another sweet intolerance, so to speak. Sucrose is sugar, commonly found in beet sugar, cane sugar, or table sugar. Because sucrose intolerance is so closely related to fructose intolerance, many people lump the two together. The causes, symptoms, and testing protocol are identical, but for people with sucrose intolerance, sucrose, not fructose, is the issue. These individuals lack an enzyme called sucrase that is needed to digest sucrose.

Most people can tolerate small amounts of sucrose, but, again, you'll have to experiment to find out what the right amount is for your body. And while there's no cure for sucrose intolerance, you can manage it by avoiding all forms of table sugar, including sugarcane, powdered sugar, brown sugar, maple syrup, and molasses.

If you haven't seen great results from tweaking your diet or you do want to eat some foods with sucrose, you can also take an enzyme supplement called Sucraid. Buy it over the counter at your local drugstore and take it with each meal. If you've forgotten to pop it, you can still take it after eating, but try to do it within thirty minutes of your meal.

A Taste of MSG

Food additives can also cause intolerances, especially one called monosodium glutamate, or MSG. MSG is a flavor enhancer, and although it's used heavily in Chinese cooking, which is why many people refer to this as Chinese restaurant syndrome, it's now widely used in many other foods, including canned vegetables, processed meats, seasonings and sauces, frozen dinners, soups and broths, and potato chips.

If you have MSG intolerance, you'll know if you've ingested some, since you might experience flushing, sensations of warmth, headaches, chest discomfort, abdominal pain, bloating, diarrhea, and nausea. Ironically, even though he grew up in China, where he frequently ate MSG, Dr. Qian developed an intolerance to MSG after he moved to the United States.

Avoiding MSG is your best bet for staying symptom-free, but because MSG is added to numerous foods, especially processed foods, cutting it from your diet can be a challenge. That's why it's important to learn how to spot MSG in food items.

The following ingredients indicate that MSG is always present:

Autolyzed yeast
Calcium caseinate
Gelatin
Glutamate
Glutamic acid
Hydrolyzed protein
Monopotassium glutamate
Monosodium glutamate
Sodium caseinate
Textured protein
Yeast extract
Yeast food
Yeast nutrient

These terms may indicate a food contains MSG:

Barley malt
Bouillon and broth
Carmageenan
Citric acid
Malt extract
Malt flavoring
Maltodextrin
Natural beef flavoring

Natural chicken flavoring

Natural pork flavoring

Pectin

Protease

Protein (fortified)

Soy protein or soy protein concentrate

Soy protein isolate

Soy sauce stock or soy sauce extract

Ultrapasteurized

Whey protein

Whey protein isolate

Whey protein concentrate

Fortunately, grocery stores now stock numerous MSG-free foods. Restaurants, even Asian-inspired ones, are also creating MSG-free dishes. Yet this doesn't guarantee that the food will be 100 percent MSG-free. Although the restaurant may not have added MSG to any of its foods, MSG could easily be hiding in an ingredient it uses.

That shouldn't stop you from going out—it never stops Dr. Qian, and on the rare occasion when he does eat MSG, he just deals with the symptoms—but you need to be aware of this in case you do have a reaction.

Sneaky Sulfite

If you're a beer or wine drinker, you're probably familiar with sulfites, since these compounds occur naturally in the process of beer and wine making. They're also naturally occurring in other foods and are often added to foods to enhance flavor and preserve freshness. Although the FDA banned the use of sulfites in fresh fruits and vegetables, they're found in a variety of cooked and processed foods. Fortunately, symptoms of sulfite intolerance are usually mild, involving rashes, headaches, and cramping.

Oddly enough, though, a small number of individuals may develop an allergy to sulfite in which their body makes IgE into sulfite, a classic sign of immediate food allergy. The evidence for this isn't definitive, but these individuals may experience wheezing and potentially even anaphylactic shock. If you experience wheezing to sulfite or any other food source, see an allergist. True allergy to sulfite, if it exists, is very rare.

To manage sulfite intolerance, avoid eating foods that contain sulfite. As with other intolerances, you'll have to get savvy about reading food labels. Look for these ingredients on food labels: sulfur dioxide, potassium bisulfite, potassium metabisulfite, sodium bisulfite, sodium metabisulfite, sodium sulfite, and anything ending in "sulfite."

To make you an even better sulfite detective, carry this list of possible sulfite-containing foods with you the next time you go to the grocery store:

- Alcoholic beverages: beer, cocktail mixes, wine, wine coolers
- Baked goods: cookies, crackers, mixes with dried fruits or vegetables, piecrust, pizza crust, quiche crust, flour tortillas
- Beverages: dried citrus-fruit beverage mixes
- Condiments and relishes: horseradish, onion and pickle relishes, pickles, olives, salad-dressing mixes, wine vinegar
- Confections/frostings: brown, raw, powdered, or white sugar derived from sugar beets
- Fish/shellfish: canned clams; fresh, frozen, or dried shrimp; frozen lobster; scallops; dried cod
- Gelatins, puddings, fillings: fruit fillings, flavored and unflavored gelatin, pectin jelling agents
- Grains and pastas: cornstarch, modified food starch, spinach pasta, gravies, hominy, breadings, batters, noodle/rice mixes
- Jams and jellies: all jams and jellies
- Nut products
- Processed fruits: canned, bottled, or frozen fruit juices (including lemon, lime, grape, and apple);

　　canned, bottled, or frozen dietetic fruit or fruit
　　juices; dried fruit; maraschino cherries; glazed
　　fruit; shredded coconut

- Processed vegetables: vegetable juice, canned vegetables, pickled vegetables, dried vegetables, instant mashed potatoes, frozen potatoes, potato salad
- Snack foods: dried fruit snacks, trail mixes, filled crackers
- Soups: canned seafood soups, dried soup mixes
- Sweet sauces, toppings: corn syrup, maple syrup, fruit toppings, high-fructose corn syrup, pancake syrup
- Tea: instant tea, liquid tea concentrates

One other note: If you have a confirmed history of wheezing from sulfite exposure, especially if you are prescribed an injected medication, ask if it is preserved with sulfite.

Terrible Tyramine

Tyramine is a substance found naturally in foods. It can also be produced in foods and beverages as a result of fermentation or aging. In fact, the longer a food ages, the higher its tyramine content is. If you have an intolerance to tyramine, headaches and migraines are two common symptoms.

As with other intolerances, avoid eating foods with tyramine. These include aged cheese; cured meats like sausage, pepperoni, and salami; sauerkraut; soy sauce; yeast-extract spreads like Marmite; fava bean pods; banana peels; draft or unpasteurized beer; and some wines.

Why Alcohol May Not Make You Happy

If you have an intolerance to alcohol, you'll know almost immediately, for the alcohol will probably cause you to have nasal congestion and a flushed face. Other symptoms include a runny or stuffy nose, rapid heartbeat, headache, nausea, vomiting, heartburn, abdominal pain, and increased problems with existing asthma.

If you're one of these individuals, you have a genetic condition in which you lack an enzyme called aldehyde dehydrogenase. As a result, your body's unable to break down alcohol. Even small amounts of alcohol will cause symptoms, so it's best to avoid alcohol completely for the rest of your life.

Saying Good-bye to Gluten

Macaroni and cheese, spaghetti, and chocolate chip cookies are some of the great comfort foods in the American diet. Yet for people with gluten intolerance, these foods will be anything but comforting.

Gluten is a protein found in wheat, rye, and barley, and it's used in numerous foods, including baked goods, pasta, pizza crust, cereal, beer, crackers, and marinades, to name only a few. If you have gluten intolerance, your body is unable to digest gluten. As a result, you develop symptoms like abdominal discomfort, flatulence, diarrhea, fatigue, and depression.

Unfortunately, there are no tests to diagnose gluten intolerance. Many people make this diagnosis on their own, but because cutting gluten from your diet can be a cumbersome task and carries significant social ramifications, we recommend that you seek medical help. You'll probably undergo a blood test to rule out immediate and delayed food allergies to wheat. If those tests don't reveal anything suspicious, you'll then be asked to eliminate gluten from your diet to see if symptoms resolve. If you feel better on this diet, it's logical to assume that you have gluten intolerance.

Because celiac disease is linked to gluten consumption, you'll also undergo testing for celiac disease,

The GCFC Diet—Could It Help Your Child's Behavioral Issues?

If you have a child with autism or another developmental disorder, you've no doubt heard about the gluten-free, casein-free (GFCF) diet. Many people believe that by removing wheat and milk protein, also known as gluten and casein, from the diet, symptoms of autism and other disorders improve.

Unfortunately, though, there's no strong research to support this theory. In fact, several studies have shown no significant benefits for children with developmental disorders who eat a GFCF diet. Imposing this diet on children could also cause nutritional deficiencies.

That's not easy information for many parents to swallow, especially because this diet is so widely accepted and supported by numerous autism groups. So what should you do? If you want to give this diet a shot—and we certainly understand that you want to do everything you can for your child—we advise doing a test run with this diet for three months. You should also consult with a nutrition specialist to make sure your child is eating the right nutrients.

During those three months, see if you spot any behavioral changes in your child. As much as we hate to say this, it's unlikely that you'll see changes, which is why most of our patients eventually abandon the GCFC diet.

which may include blood testing and an endoscopy. Don't think, though, that having gluten intolerance means you have celiac disease. Although people often confuse the two conditions, they are different.

People who have celiac disease must follow a strict, lifelong gluten-free diet, or they can suffer serious health consequences. With gluten intolerance, however, you can often tolerate small amounts of gluten. If you do eat more than you can handle, you might feel sick for a day, but your symptoms aren't life-threatening and will resolve as soon as the gluten passes through you.

Of course, this leads to an obvious question: Can gluten intolerance lead to celiac disease? Although we can't offer a definitive answer, it's possible but unlikely. There's also no evidence to suggest that if celiac disease has been ruled out, you're doing damage to your intestines by continuing to eat gluten.

Dietary changes are the best way to manage gluten intolerance. You may not have to cut all gluten from your diet, but you'll have to experiment to know what your body can handle.

Follow these tips to avoid gluten:

- Give up foods with grains that contain gluten, including wheat, rye, and barley. Instead, choose these alternatives: rice, corn, soy, potato, tapioca, beans, garfava flour, sorghum, quinoa, millet, buckwheat, arrowroot, amaranth, teff flour, Montina, and nut flours.

- Avoid cross-contamination. If you're living with somebody who doesn't have gluten intolerance, their gluten-containing products could contaminate your gluten-free foods. For instance, your gluten-free bread could pick up wheat crumbs in the toaster or that peanut butter your wife uses to slather on her wheat bread could contain wheat crumbs. Keep these items separate as much as you can.

- Keep an eye on oats. Oats have sparked a lot of controversy, largely because they can be contaminated or tainted with gluten. Yet for most gluten-intolerant individuals, the amount of contamination is so minute that they're able to eat oats without problems. If, though, you have celiac disease, you'll need to make sure that any oats you eat haven't been processed in a plant that also processes wheat, barley, and rye.

- Read food labels. Dozens of processed foods contain gluten, including salad dressings, pudding mixes, canned soups, tortilla chips, luncheon meats, and flavored and frozen yogurt. Gluten often hides under other names, too, making it tough to spot. If you see any of these terms, gluten is present: barley, malt, malt flavoring, malt vinegar, rye, triticale, and wheat (durum, graham, kamut, semolina, spelt).

- Look for gluten-free foods and restaurants with gluten-free options. There's never been a better time to have gluten intolerance, since numerous restaurants now offer gluten-free menus. You can also find dozens of gluten-free food products in grocery stores. Just remember, though, that food manufacturers often change their ingredients, so don't get lazy about reading food labels, even if you've been eating a product for years.

- Say cheers wisely. If you'd like to sip a cocktail, know that wine is gluten-free. However, unless you're drinking a gluten-free kind, beers, ales, and lagers are made from grains that contain gluten.

- Check for gluten in your medications. Medications frequently contain gluten, which is why you should ask your pharmacist. To be extra sure, call the manufacturer.

- Get savvy about nonfood items. Self-stick labels, lickable envelopes, rubber gloves, art supplies, lipstick, shampoos, sunscreen, soaps, skin lotions, toothpaste, and mouthwash may also contain gluten.

Then, follow this chart to know what you can and can't eat:

Food group:	Foods to eat:	Foods to avoid:
Cereal products, flours, baking products	Arrowroot, corn flour, cornmeal, polenta, rice flour, potato flour, soy flour, lentil flour, millet, rice (brown, white, wild), sago, tapioca, buckwheat, amaranth, quinoa, baby rice cereal, rice bran, psyllium, soy-based lecithin, rice and corn breakfast cereals, homemade or commercial muesli using allowed ingredients, gluten-free pasta made with allowed flours, rice vermicelli, custard	Wheat; wheat starch; wheat-based corn flour; semolina; rye flour; triticale; bulgur; couscous; wheat germ; wheat bran; oat bran; barley; oats produced in a plant that also manufactures gluten, malt, malt extract, maltodextrin, wheat, or mixed grain breakfast cereal; pasta; puddings and custard powders made from unsuitable flours; icing sugar mixtures; thickener (unless you check with manufacturer);

Food group:	Foods to eat:	Foods to avoid:
	powder (check ingredients), glucose, dextrose, caramel, sugar (brown, white, and raw), pure icing sugar, gelatin	pregel starch; starch; modified starch (unless sources are checked)
Vegetables, fruits, legumes, nuts, and seeds	Fresh, frozen, dried, or canned vegetables and fruits without sauce; vegetable and fruit juice; dried beans; canned beans (check ingredients); nuts and seeds; peanut butter; tofu	Canned or frozen vegetables in sauce; vegetarian products including textured vegetable protein; commercially thickened fruit-pie fillings; fruit pies with wheat-based pastry; tofu burgers; beer nuts; baked beans (check ingredients)

(continued)

Food group:	Foods to eat:	Foods to avoid:
Meat, fish, poultry, and soups	Fresh, smoked, and corned meat, fish, and poultry; any foods in this group that are frozen without sauce, crumbs, or batter; canned meat or fish without sauce; ham off bone; bacon; corned beef; gluten-free sausages; eggs; tofu; homemade soups from gluten-free ingredients; some commercial soups (check ingredients); homemade pizzas using allowed ingredients	Meat and fish prepared or thickened with flour, batter, or breadcrumbs; flavored tunas (check ingredients); egg sausage; processed meats; meat pies and sausage rolls; frozen dinners; tofu burgers; homemade or commercial soups made with thickeners, stocks, pasta, barley, or flours containing gluten; commercial pizzas

Food group:	Foods to eat:	Foods to avoid:
Dairy products, butter, margarine, and oil	Full cream and low-fat milks; evaporated, powdered, and condensed milk; buttermilk; yogurt and other ice cream (check ingredients); block, processed cream and cottage cheese; milk flavoring if malt- and gluten-free; malt-free soy milk and those labeled gluten-free; butter, margarine, and oils	Malted milk; milk flavorings; artificial cream; ice cream thickeners or flavorings that contain gluten; ice cream cones and waffles; cheese mixtures; pastas and spreads unless checked; soy milk with malt
Condiments and other flavorings	Balsamic, cider, red wine, and white vinegar;	Malt vinegar; commercial mustards, salad dressings, *(continued)*

Food group:	Foods to eat:	Foods to avoid:
	some commercial mustards and salad dressings; some sauces, pickles, relishes, and chutneys; soy sauce (check ingredients); Tabasco sauce; gluten-free stock powders; curry paste and powder (check ingredients); gluten-free gravy; tomato pastes; tahini; fresh and dried herbs and spices; jam, honey, peanut, and other nut butters; pure maple and golden syrup; plain and	sauces, pickles, relishes, chutneys and salsas (unless checked); barbecue salts and other flavoring mixes; yeast extract

Food group:	Foods to eat:	Foods to avoid:
	flavored gelatin; cocoa; flavoring essences and artificial sweeteners (check ingredients)	
Beverages	Water, milk, tea, coffee, cordials, soft drinks (including diet), mineral water, cocoa, drinking chocolate (check ingredients), wine, sherry, whiskey, bourbon, vodka, rum, tequila	Coffee substitutes, chocolate milk flavorings, barley-based cordial, beer, ale, stout, vermouth, gin
Snacks	Plain corn and potato chips; popcorn	Some flavored snacks like corn chips; filled chocolates (check ingredients); licorice

Fact or Fiction: Going Gluten-Free Will Help You Lose Weight

Want to lose weight? Go gluten-free. Or so the latest diet trend advocates. Yet can you really lose weight on a gluten-free diet? It's possible, but not because there's anything magical about cutting gluten.

The main source of gluten is wheat, which is found in many of America's favorite high-carbohydrate, high-calorie foods, including pizza, pretzels, cookies, cakes, and bread. Because you've now limited your food choices, many of which are laden with fat and calories, it stands to reason that you could drop some weight.

Just beware: Gluten-free doesn't mean calorie-free or fat-free. Some gluten-free foods contain more carbs, sugar, fat, and calories and less nutrients than their regular counterparts, which could send the scale zooming in the other direction.

Our advice? Cut gluten only if you have gluten intolerance or celiac disease. Otherwise, lose that weight by eating a healthy, balanced diet and exercising regularly.

Sizing Up Celiac Disease

No doubt you've been hearing a lot about celiac disease lately. Here's why: A study published in 2010 found that celiac disease increased fivefold during a fifteen-year period, especially among the elderly. While this once rare disease has always been thought to be primarily genetic, researchers in this study found that environmental factors caused the immune system to lose its tolerance to gluten.

Today, celiac disease, which is also called celiac sprue, gluten sensitive enteropathy, and nontropical sprue, affects about one of out 133 individuals, according to the Celiac Disease Foundation. Even more alarming? Roughly 97 percent of people with celiac disease go undiagnosed, which could wreak havoc on your health.

Although anybody can develop celiac disease, people at higher risk for the disease include those with type 1 diabetes, autoimmune thyroid disease, a skin disease called dermatitis herpetiformis, Down syndrome, Turner syndrome, or Williams syndrome. People who have a relative with celiac disease are also at greater risk for developing it.

So just what is celiac disease? It's a permanent, autoimmune response to the food protein gluten. Note, though, that it's not a food allergy, since it doesn't have the same immunological response as food allergies. Food allergies aren't autoimmune reactions, but because celiac disease does involve the immune system, it's not a food intolerance. However, we've included celiac disease in this section because it's closely related and often confused with gluten intolerance.

When people who have celiac disease eat foods with gluten, their immune system responds abnormally to the gluten by damaging fingerlike projections called villi that line the small intestine. The damaged villi are then unable to absorb basic nutrients.

Symptoms of celiac disease vary from one person to another. Ironically, people with mild versions of celiac disease may not have any symptoms. Yet classic symptoms of celiac disease in adults include abdominal cramping, intestinal gas, distention and bloating of the stomach, chronic diarrhea or constipation (or both), steatorrhea (fatty stools), anemia, or unexplained weight loss, even with a large appetite. Infants, toddlers, and young children may experience vomiting, bloated abdomen, behavioral changes, and poor growth.

Surprisingly, there are also other symptoms, many of which don't involve the gastrointestinal system. These include dental enamel defects, osteopenia, osteoporosis, bone or joint pain, fatigue, weakness, lack of energy, infertility (in men and women), depression, mouth ulcers, delayed puberty, tingling or numbness in the hands or feet, elevated liver enzymes, and migraine headaches.

Left untreated, celiac disease can cause nutritional and immune-related disorders. According to the Celiac Disease Foundation, long-term conditions resulting from untreated celiac disease include type I diabetes, hypothyroidism, rheumatoid arthritis, iron deficiency anemia, early onset osteoporosis or osteopenia, vitamin K deficiency (associated with risk for hemorrhaging), vitamin and mineral deficiencies, central and peripheral nervous system disorders, pancreatic insufficiency, intestinal lymphomas and other gastrointestinal cancers, gallbladder malfunction, and neurological manifestations.

If you suspect that you have celiac disease, you shouldn't cut gluten from your diet until you've undergone testing. In fact, it's generally recommended that you eat gluten for at least four weeks for the most accurate test results. As mentioned in the previous chapter, the two most common tests are blood tests and endoscopy.

Genetic testing is also available, although know that this doesn't diagnose celiac disease and doctors won't routinely order it. Instead, individuals usually undergo this testing to satisfy their curiosity. The test determines whether you have two genes, HLA DQ2 and DQ8, which are necessary for celiac disease to develop. Roughly one-third of the population carries these genes, so having them doesn't guarantee that you'll develop celiac disease. Instead, it indicates that you could develop celiac disease. On the flip side, if you don't have these genes, you can be certain that you won't develop celiac disease.

If you are diagnosed with celiac disease, the only treatment is to follow a gluten-free diet for the rest of your life, since you can never outgrow this condition. We can't stress this enough, because any amount of gluten, even what you might consider a miniscule amount, can cause health problems. We've treated individuals, in fact, who have been diagnosed with celiac disease but have ignored our warning to avoid gluten completely; they've then developed serious health conditions.

So how do you remove gluten from your diet? Check out the above section on gluten intolerance for this information. Dietitians and support groups can also help you make the transition to a gluten-free life.

As you start this diet, you should also remove lactose from your diet (see the lactose intolerance section in this chapter), since you can develop temporary lactose intolerance. Once the villi are regenerated, however, lactose intolerance usually disappears.

Because celiac disease can affect your bone health, you'll also have to undergo a DEXA bone-density test when you receive your diagnosis. Children with celiac disease, some of whom have delayed bone age, will need

Fighting the Food-Dye Myth

Food dyes don't have it easy these days: They've been vili-fied by numerous individuals who claim they cause food in-tolerances and food allergies and blame their rashes, face flushing, even behavioral changes in kids on food dyes. The truth? Although many people suspect they have adverse re-actions to dyes, we know of only a couple of dyes that cause food allergy. The most widly reported is due to a protein called cochineal that's derived from crushed beetle carcasses and used in red dye. Another comes from the annatto seed, which is used for yellow or orange coloring. In both cases, these are natural dyes that have protein and as we've already learned, proteins are what the immune system predominantly responds to. Most dyes, in contrast, are very small molecules that are not potent inducers of im-mune (i.e., allergic) responses. There's also no reliable data that we know of to support the idea that food dyes alter behavior in children.

to undergo a different test called a bone-age study, which is an X-ray of the left hand. If the test indicates low bone-mineral density, you'll undergo another test twelve months later.

In addition, you should wear a medical alert bracelet in case you're ever in a situation where you become unconscious; you should wear this bracelet all the time, even at home. (Contact the MedicAlert Foundation at www.medicalert.org or 888-633-4298 to purchase a bracelet.) The bracelet should disclose that you have celiac disease and include emergency contact information.

Finally, you'll need to have a blood test every year to make sure the gluten-free diet is working and that you haven't developed any autoimmune diseases like hypothyroidism or diabetes.

Although celiac disease is a serious condition, here's the good news: Once you remove gluten from your diet, your small intestine will begin to heal, and your overall health will improve. Symptoms generally improve within two to four weeks of following this diet. Six to twelve months later, all of your symptoms will be gone, and the lining of your intestine will have healed.

part III

Food Allergies

chapter 6

Let's Evaluate Your Symptoms

As we've suggested, food allergies are less mysterious than food intolerances. Of course, we still don't know everything about food allergies, but suffice it to say that food allergies are much less mysterious than food intolerances.

For people who have a food allergy, this will probably come as only slightly comforting news, for living with a food allergy can be scary. After all, food allergies can lead to anaphylaxis, a severe allergic reaction, or even death. In an ideal world, we'd be able to identify those people who are at greatest risk, but we're not there yet.

Fortunately, though, the combination of avoiding trigger foods and getting prompt emergency treatment is highly effective in combating food allergy reactions. While it's true that from 2001 to 2005 an average of 90,000 visits were made each year to emergency rooms for food-allergic reactions, the Centers for Disease Control and Prevention estimates that there are only 150 deaths from food allergies each year. In our opinion, that's still 150 too many, but it does mean that given the more than 10 million people who have food allergies, your individual risk of the worst-case scenario is low.

Food allergies certainly are serious, but the more you learn about your food allergy, the less scary it will be, and the more you can enjoy life and food. Let's take a closer look at food allergies.

Do These Scenarios Sound Familiar?

If you think food allergies are all about hives and rashes and other immediate symptoms, you might be in for a surprise. While it's true that those are classic and common symptoms of food allergies, food allergies can cause other problems, and some of them, like difficulty swallowing meat, are the result of chronic inflammation rather than an immediate type of response.

To show you how different food allergies can look, we'd like you to meet four individuals, each of whom has a different set of problems. As you read these four case studies, see if any of them sound familiar.

Case Study #1: *Elizabeth*
The problem: *Itchy mouth and swollen lip after eating*

Elizabeth has battled seasonal allergies for years. She also has exercise-induced asthma, and last year, at the age of thirty-nine, began to experience odd symptoms. After eating fresh (but never cooked) fruits like apples, peaches, plums, and cherries, her gums and lips would often itch and swell. Although the swelling was mild, it was annoying and somewhat embarrassing, especially when she was with friends or work colleagues.

A month ago, the same thing happened when she ate only a small amount of a strawberry-almond smoothie. She was frustrated enough to call her family physician, who advised her to avoid all nuts. Even though Elizabeth has eaten peanuts, cashews, and walnuts many times in the past, she began following her doctor's advice. She decided to avoid strawberries, too, just in case.

Her doctor also recommended doing a blood test to determine if she had any food allergies. Those tests revealed that Elizabeth was strongly positive to birch and moderately positive to almond, hazelnut, and peach. The end diagnosis? A food allergy known as oral allergy syndrome.

Today, Elizabeth eats all nuts, with the exception

of hazelnuts, which cause the same symptoms as the fruits. She also avoids any fruits that bother her, especially when her seasonal allergies are at their worst. Luckily, she's not at high risk for anaphylaxis and doesn't need to carry an epinephrine autoinjector or take any other precautions for her allergy.

Case study #2: *Nathan*
The problem: *Eczema in an infant*

When Nathan was two months old, he developed rashes. They started as patches of dry and sometimes inflamed skin on his torso and progressed to include more of his body, including his hands, face, and head. They were worse in the folds of his skin, which Nathan often scratched until they bled. During the worst outbreaks, he had trouble sleeping at night, so his parents would give him Benadryl.

When Nathan first developed rashes, he was eating a milk-based formula without solid foods. His parents introduced solid foods to him at five months old, starting with rice, oats, sweet potatoes, green beans, apples, peaches, and pears. Yet because Nathan's parents thought his condition got worse when they introduced wheat, they began limiting it in his diet.

Suspicious that Nathan had food allergies, his doctor referred him to an allergist who performed skin testing for wheat, soy, egg, peanut, and milk when Nathan was eight months old. Although wheat was negative, Nathan did test positive in varying degrees for the others, suggesting that he might be allergic to those foods.

Nathan's doctor recommended treating his eczema first, using a topical steroid and regular moisturizer. Because the rash improved with this standard treatment, Nathan's doctor recommended not restricting anything from his diet that he was regularly consuming, including milk.

Over the next few months, Nathan was tested at various times to foods that were either suspected to be a problem (like wheat) or foods he hadn't yet eaten but were positive on the skin test. The allergist used a food challenge, and Nathan passed everything but peanuts.

Although peanut allergies are tough to outgrow, Nathan's doctor is hopeful he can eventually eat peanuts, but has advised his parents to keep all peanuts out of his diet until he's tested again, perhaps at four years old. He also prescribed an epinephrine autoinjector and gave Nathan's parents an emergency action plan in case of accidental ingestion and information about food labels.

Case study #3: Jonathan
The problem: Trouble swallowing after eating
beef or chicken

Twenty-six-year-old Jonathan has been healthy his
entire life. However, for the past ten months, he's been
having trouble swallowing when eating. Food just feels
like it's getting stuck in his throat. At first, he thought
maybe he wasn't chewing properly. Yet even with more
conscious chewing, the problem has persisted to a point
where he's had to cut his food into food miniscule pieces
and drink lots of liquid to wash it down, especially if
it's steak or chicken.

A recent incident, though, prompted medical attention. Jonathan was at a restaurant with friends when he
began to choke and cough violently on a piece of steak.
His friend performed the Heimlich maneuver on him,
but when that didn't work, Jonathan was rushed to the
emergency room by ambulance.

He was seen by a gastroenterologist, who performed
an endoscopy. Sure enough, there was a piece of meat
stuck in Jonathan's esophagus, which the doctor removed. His esophagus also looked inflamed, and bi-
opsies revealed esophagitis, an inflammation of the
esophagus.

After taking an antacid medicine for two months,
Jonathan felt better but still had some swallowing dif-

ficulties. When Jonathan returned to the gastroenterologist for another endoscopy, the doctor diagnosed him
with eosinophilic esophagitis, a condition often caused
by food allergies. He then saw an allergist and had blood
and skin allergy testing, which suggested that he may
be allergic to beef and chicken.

Next, Jonathan went on an elimination diet for eight
weeks, avoiding beef, chicken, and a few other common
allergens. At the end of the eight weeks, he underwent a
biopsy, which showed that he had no inflammation,
meaning that his condition had resolved.

With that diagnosis in hand, he began to gradually reintroduce foods back to his diet and learned that
milk and chicken were the culprits. Later, he revealed
that according to his mother, he had a lot of trouble
as an infant with milk-based formula and didn't drink
much milk as a toddler or young child. Whether the two
are related is unclear, but as long as Jonathan avoids
milk and chicken, he won't have any problems.

Case study #4: *Claire*
The problem: *Bloody stools in an otherwise
happy, growing child*

Two-month-old Claire has been fed with breast milk
exclusively since birth. She's been gaining weight well,
but ever since she was two weeks old, her mother has

noticed specks of blood in her stools. This worry prompted her to take Claire to the pediatrician.

The pediatrician found nothing out of the ordinary, but she was concerned about the bloody stools and sent Claire to a pediatric gastroenterologist for further evaluation. Tests revealed that Claire may have allergic colitis, a form of delayed food allergy.

Since then, because she's breast-feeding Claire, her mother has eliminated all dairy from her own diet. As a result, Claire's bloody stools have gradually resolved. Her mother was also advised not to give Claire any dairy until she turns one, at which point she can try to introduce it back into her diet.

Did any of those four scenarios sound familiar? If you identified with one of the first two situations, it's possible you have what's called an immediate food allergy. If, however, one of the last two scenarios sounded more like what you're going through, you or your child could have a delayed food allergy.

So what does all of this mean? Let's take a closer look at each type of allergy so you can get a better handle on what you might be facing.

What You Should Know About Immediate Food Allergies

Ask people to name the most common symptoms of a food allergy, and most would probably list rashes, hives, and wheezing. They're not wrong, but what they've identified is one of two categories of food allergies that we call immediate food allergies. It's the most common type of food allergy, affecting anywhere from 2 percent to 5 percent of the population.

As you might expect, immediate food allergies are so named because symptoms can begin within a few minutes up to a few hours of eating an offending food. In severe but rare cases, you don't even have to eat the food. Just touching it or breathing in particles of that food could trigger a response. Yet the risk for dangerously severe reactions from touching the allergen to the skin is minimal.

Why, though, does the body respond in such an abnormal way to food? Blame an immunoglobin in your body called IgE.

First, though, a primer on the immune system: As you know, your immune system is designed to protect you against foreign agents and infectious organisms. To do that, it produces four different classes of antibodies: IgG, IgA, IgM, and IgE. (Ig, by the way, stands for immunoglobin, while the letter after Ig designates the particular antibody.) All of these antibodies strengthen the immune system, but it's IgE, which is mostly bound to specialized immune cells in the lungs, skin, and mucous membranes, that induces allergic reactions against foreign substances. That's why immediate food allergies are also referred to as IgE-mediated food allergies.

The first time your immune system is exposed to a potential allergen, you won't experience any allergic reaction. That's because your body has to make an IgE response before you can have an allergic reaction. Yet you don't have to eat the allergen; your immune system might be exposed by another route, possibly before you were even born.

What you don't realize, though, is that your body has already sprung into action, producing a specific IgE antibody to certain allergens in that food. (You can be allergic to more than one food, but with rare exceptions of highly similar and thus cross-reactive allergens, the IgE antibodies have to match that food allergen exactly. If you're allergic to several foods, your body will produce IgE antibodies for the allergens in each food.) Those IgE antibodies circulate through your body and attach to basophils in the blood and mast cells in body tissues, especially in your nose, throat, lungs, skin, and gastrointestinal tract. Doctors refer to this first response as sensitization, meaning that your body has begun the process of producing IgE antibodies to a food.

When you eat the food again, the allergen in that food now comes in contact with the IgE antibodies, which are bound to mast cells and basophils. That interaction signals those cells to release histamine and other chemicals, which cause the symptoms of allergic reactions.

Symptoms can vary widely—you might even respond differently to the same food on different days—and can involve multiple organ systems or be limited to only one of those systems. The symptoms you experience will depend in part on which tissues these chemicals are released in. Here are some of the most common symptoms with immediate food allergies:

- Respiratory tract: wheezing, coughing, hoarse voice, breathing difficulty, runny and/or itchy nose, sneezing
- Skin: hives, swelling (called angiodema), itchiness, flushing, flaring of eczema
- Gastrointestinal tract: nausea, vomiting, abdominal cramps, diarrhea

The severity of these symptoms can also fluctuate, depending on the amount of the offending food you've eaten and other factors. Those other factors might

Forbidden Fruits (and Veggies)—The Scoop on Oral Allergy Syndrome

You love chomping fresh fruits and veggies, even various nuts. Trouble is, every time you eat a certain food like hazelnuts or apples, you get an itchy mouth and swollen lips. Sometimes the swelling is dramatic. Your throat often feels itchy or tight, too. Could you have a food allergy? Yes, but this type of immediate food allergy actually starts as a pollen allergy.

What you're experiencing is a condition called oral allergy syndrome, also called pollen-related or pollen-food-allergy syndrome. In people who have allergies to pollen (like trees, grass, weeds, and plants), the immune system recognizes a similarity between the proteins of pollen and those in food, which is sufficient to trigger a reaction. Symptoms usually occur within minutes of eating the food. While most people who have this syndrome struggle with it year-round, others may only have problems during the season that their pollen allergies are active.

Yet don't think you're destined to develop oral allergy syndrome just because you have seasonal allergies. Not everybody who has seasonal allergies will experience this syndrome. There is a weak relation between the severity of seasonal allergies and risk of developing oral allergy syndrome, but, for the most part, we don't know why people develop this condition. In fact, some of Dr. Wayne's patients have very mild seasonal symptoms, even though they have a strong sensitization to pollen and experience symptoms when eating certain plant foods.

Fortunately, reactions from oral allergy syndrome are rarely dangerous and usually resolve within twenty to thirty minutes, even without treatment. Generally, though, you can quell symptoms with medication like an over-the-counter antihistamine, including the newer, nonsedating type called cetirizine.

Although you can deal with this problem on your own, you can also work with an allergist, who can confirm that you have oral allergy syndrome and not a more serious allergy, especially if you experience symptoms with peanuts or tree nuts. In fact, there's now a test to determine whether you're allergic solely to the pollen-related protein in peanuts and tree nuts or the protein in the peanut or tree nuts that's not related to pollen. If it's the latter, which would indicate a more serious form of food allergy, the allergist would recommend that you carry epinephrine. However, for the former, which is oral allergy syndrome, your reactions are unlikely to be severe, and you'll probably be advised to avoid the offending foods, although recommendations will vary.

(continued)

There's also mixed evidence that allergy shots for the pollens may decrease symptoms of oral allergy syndrome. However, because this treatment hasn't been proven to treat oral allergy syndrome, it's not recommended for this condition alone.

The good news is that oral allergy syndrome can change throughout life. Although it usually develops in adolescence or early adulthood and typically sticks around for most of adulthood, it can become less severe with age. Pregnancy can also decrease (or in some cases, increase) symptoms.

To manage this condition, learn what foods cross-react with the pollen you're allergic to. If you have an allergy to birch-tree pollen, you'll most likely have a reaction to apples, peaches, pears, plums, cherries, hazelnuts, almonds, and, less often, other fruits and vegetables. If, though, ragweed triggers your allergies, you may react to banana, kiwi, melons (i.e., watermelon, honeydew, and cantaloupe), and occasionally other plants.

Then avoid those foods that give you symptoms, especially during your allergy season. Eating cooked forms of these foods, however, should present no problem. The allergens in these foods are sensitive to heat, so even just a few seconds in the microwave is enough to alter them so they don't cause reactions. Peeling the skin, which often contains more allergens than the meat of the fruit, can also help.

include preexisting asthma, especially if it's poorly controlled; eating the allergen on an empty stomach; a concurrent illness; other allergic exposure; or eating the food along with exercising or drinking alcohol.

The most severe symptom is anaphylaxis, which can lead to death if not treated immediately. We'll discuss anaphylaxis in greater detail in the next chapter.

Meet the Common Culprits Behind Immediate Food Allergies

When you consider how many foods are in the American diet, it's amazing that only eight cause the most problems. That's not to say you can't develop an immediate food allergy to almost any food (with the exception of foods that have no proteins). Yet there are eight allergens in particular that account for 90 percent of all food allergies. (For tips on how to avoid these allergens, turn to chapter 8.)

Pesky Peanuts

Peanut butter and jelly sandwiches are as American as apple pie. What kid, after all, didn't grow up on this staple? Turns out, slightly more than 1 percent of kids won't be able to participate in this American pastime, for their peanut allergy will stop them. This number is actually on the rise, as one study found that peanut allergies in children nearly tripled between 1997 and 2008.

Peanut allergies are considered one of the most dangerous, largely because peanuts, even trace amounts, can cause severe reactions. And although about 20 percent of children outgrow this allergy, this will be a lifelong struggle for the remaining 80 percent. Another compounding factor? Roughly 30 percent to 40 percent of children who have a peanut allergy also have a tree nut allergy, which is why they're sometimes advised to avoid tree nuts, too.

Yet there is some encouraging news about peanut allergies: Just touching or inhaling the scent of peanuts is unlikely to cause a systemic reaction. In one study, 100 percent of thirty peanut-allergic children who had skin contact with peanut butter only developed hives, while those who smelled peanut butter developed no symptoms.

Instead, accidental ingestion is the biggest concern with this allergy. For instance, maybe your peanut-allergic child eats an egg roll that was sealed using peanut butter without declaring it, or a baker uses the same spatula to prepare two cookie batters, one with peanuts and one that's not supposed to contain any peanuts.

That's why alerting caregivers about your child's peanut allergy and reading food labels are essential. If you see a warning label that a particular food product may contain nuts, take it seriously. Just because you or your child has tolerated a food with a label like that in the past, there's no guarantee there won't be sufficient contamination to cause a reaction next time.

Going Out on a Limb for Tree Nuts

It should be no surprise that tree nuts—almonds, Brazil nuts, cashews, hazelnuts, macadamia nuts, pecans, pistachios, and walnuts—grow on trees. (Peanuts, by the way, grow in the soil.) Although tree nuts aren't in the same family as peanuts, some of their allergens are similar, which may be why many people with peanut allergies have tree nut allergies, too. People can also be allergic to more than one tree nut. And, like peanut allergies, tree nut allergies are rarely outgrown; only about 9 percent of children with this allergy outgrow it.

Just as with peanut allergies, a small amount of tree nuts can cause reactions, some of which can be severe. Yet it's that accidental ingestion you need to worry about most.

So does this mean you should avoid all tree nuts if you have a tree nut allergy? Not necessarily. In fact, eating tree nuts you're not allergic to could help reduce your risk of ever becoming allergic to them. It might also help you feel more normal if you know you can eat some tree nuts. If you decide to go this route, just be aware of high-risk situations and areas of cross-contamination, where you can't be as confident that a food doesn't contain the tree nut you're allergic to.

You should also be aware that certain tree nuts tend to cross-react more strongly with other tree nuts. For instance, pistachios and cashews are strongly cross-reactive, meaning that if you're allergic to one, you'll probably be allergic to the other. Pecans, hazelnuts, and walnuts are also cross-reactive, although less so than the pistachios and cashews.

Also, birch pollen is associated with oral allergy syndrome to almonds, hazelnuts, and, to a lesser extent, the other nuts. As previously mentioned, oral symptoms with those nuts, especially if they occur in older children and adults and exist along with seasonal allergies, warrant investigation.

If, however, you want to avoid all tree nuts, we certainly support this decision, especially if the individual with a tree nut allergy is young.

Milking It

Getting a milk mustache may not seem so appealing to the 2.5 percent of children under three who suffer from milk allergy, the most common childhood food allergy.

Sensitivity varies widely, but, as discussed above, even a person's own sensitivity may vary. While some children have a mild reaction after consuming a moderate amount of milk, others have a severe reaction after just a small amount of milk. And although hives, rashes, and itchiness are common responses from ingesting milk, vomiting and diarrhea can also occur.

Fortunately, though, 80 percent of these children outgrow the allergy by the time they're sixteen years old. For the others, this allergy can persist into adulthood, and reactions in adults tend to be severe.

Just don't confuse a milk allergy with lactose intolerance. While lactose-intolerant individuals have symptoms because of the sugar in milk, people with milk allergies react to one or more of the main milk proteins like lactoglobulin or the caseins.

So if you have a milk allergy, should you avoid all milk products? Surprisingly, we've noticed that some individuals with milk allergy who react to fresh forms of milk tolerate milk protein as an ingredient in baked goods. Researchers have recently discovered that for these children, there appears to be no harm—and may even be some benefit—in manipulating the diet to include those foods if they can tolerate them.

The Bad Egg

Your child may eat up Dr. Seuss, but if an egg allergy is lurking, make sure his or her real diet doesn't include any of those green eggs (or any color, for that matter!). Egg allergy is the second most common food allergy in children, but the good news is that most outgrow them. In fact, by the age of sixteen, 68 percent of kids have outgrown this allergy.

Because allergens live in the egg white, many egg-allergic individuals think they can eat the yolk without any problem. Yet the yolk can easily be contaminated with allergens, so avoid the entire egg. Also, while hens' eggs pose the most problems, other bird eggs might also cause a reaction, so you should avoid them as well.

An added problem with an egg allergy is that egg hides in a great many products, which is why you need to read food labels carefully. Yet like a milk allergy, some individuals can tolerate egg in baked products, and studies suggest no harm if these individuals eat them. Ask your allergist if a baked-egg test might be worth trying.

Two other points we want to address about egg allergies: You might have heard that egg allergy is associated with an increased risk of asthma, which you may think means that one causes the other, which is not entirely true. It is true that all children with food allergy have an increased risk of developing asthma. Yet an egg allergy poses the same—not greater—risk for asthma as any other food allergy.

Many families are also mistakenly instructed not to give their egg-allergic child the measles-mumps-rubella (MMR) vaccine because it contains egg. Several studies have found, however, that the MMR vaccine is safe for even the most egg-sensitive children and per recommendations from the leading allergy and pediatric medicine associations, should be given routinely by a pediatrician to children who have an egg allergy.

The flu shot, on the other hand, is slightly different. Today's flu shots contain much lower amounts of egg protein than earlier vaccines did, which is why they can be more easily given to most egg-allergic children. In fact, the CDC now recommends that unless individuals have a history of severe reactions to egg (e.g., low blood pressure, wheezing, vomiting), they may be vaccinated with the most widely administered form of the vaccine, though a history of mild reactions does indicate a longer observational period. Some people (usually children) may have a diagnosis of egg allergy, but no history of ever ingesting egg. Those individuals should consult with their allergist or other primary care doctor.

Not So Sweet Wheat

Wheat is everywhere in the American diet, making this a tough allergy to manage. Yet it usually doesn't stick around long, as the majority of kids outgrow it in childhood.

Of course, wheat allergy is sometimes confused with gluten intolerance and celiac disease, and while all three of these conditions are responses to a protein in wheat, the three are different. Usually, you can spot the difference by gauging how quickly the individual has symptoms to wheat.

Like the other immediate food allergies we're discussing, wheat allergy is distinguished by characteristic symptoms, namely that the reaction occurs within minutes to a couple of hours and is confirmed with skin or blood testing.

Soy What?

Soy is another allergen that mainly affects children, but, fortunately, most outgrow this allergy early in life.

The biggest challenge with this allergy is avoiding soy, which is found almost everywhere in the American diet.

Know, though, that many soy allergies are misdiagnosed. Perhaps because of problems with cross-reactivity with peanuts during testing, there's actually a higher rate of false positives for soy than for other food allergies. In other words, test results could reveal that you have IgE to soy even if you've never had a reaction to soy, but this doesn't mean you have a soy allergy. That's why it's crucial to work with an allergist who can interpret these tests and perform additional testing (such as a food challenge) if necessary.

Go Fish

Fish might be a nutritional powerhouse for your heart and brain, but if you have a fish allergy, going on a no-fish diet will be your ticket to health. For some reason, fish allergens stimulate the immune system to a greater degree than other allergens. Fish allergy, like that to nuts and shellfish, often persists into adulthood, making it one of the most common adult food allergies.

Because fish tends to be fairly cross-reactive, if you're allergic to one fish, you're probably going to be allergic to others. In fact, about half of the people who are allergic to one type of fish are allergic to another. If you've had a reaction that you suspect is related to fish, avoid all fish until you've been tested. Depending on the test results, you may be able to eat certain kinds of fish. For instance, you might be allergic to most white flaky fish but not tuna or salmon.

Also, because the FDA doesn't regulate fish oil as a supplement, you should probably avoid fish oil. The oil may contain enough of the protein allergens to cause problems.

A Shell of an Allergy

Shellfish is another allergy that persists into or sometimes occurs in adulthood. It's actually the most common food allergy reported by adults and usually sticks with you for life. Reactions also tend to be severe.

Shellfish are divided into two groups—crustacea and mollusks—and if you're allergic to one group, you might be able to eat some from the other group. Crustacea include shrimp, crab, and lobster, while mollusks include clams, oysters, mussels, and scallops. Until you've undergone testing with an allergist, though, avoid all shellfish.

Sesame Seeds, an Allergen on the Rise

Sesame seed allergy is common in the Middle East and Mediterranean countries, and although only about 0.1 percent of the American population is allergic to sesame seeds, sesame seed allergy may be on the rise in the United States. Some studies have found that individuals who have tree nut or peanut allergies are at increased risk of having a sesame seed allergy. Sesame seeds are frequently used in bakery and bread products, foods that naturally contain sesame seeds (i.e., hummus,

Could You Be Allergic to Exercise?

As crazy as this sounds, exercise could cause an allergic reaction, but don't think this gives you permission to be a couch potato. You just have to learn what not to eat before you exercise.

So what's going on? There's a rare condition called exercise-induced food allergy, also known as food-dependent, exercise-induced anaphylaxis, but unlike other food allergies, it requires exercise to stoke the flames, so to speak.

(continued)

Individuals who experience exercise-induced food allergy have developed an IgE antibody to an allergen in a particular food or foods. Yet only when they eat the food and then exercise do they run into trouble. In other words, they can eat the food without any problems when they're not exercising, but as soon as they combine the two, they have a reaction. Symptoms may include itching, light-headedness, hives, drop in blood pressure, even anaphylaxis. Although this could happen with many different foods, surveys indicate that wheat and celery are the most common troublemakers.

Why exercise triggers this reaction in the presence of these foods isn't exactly clear. There's speculation that exercise causes greater intestinal absorption of the food protein. As a result, a higher concentration of this protein circulates through the body and eventually contacts the mast cells and basophils, which then respond.

If this sounds familiar, work with an allergist to determine which food or foods you're allergic to. You might also have to do a food challenge and then run (or walk) on a treadmill to prove the diagnosis. The allergist will probably also prescribe epinephrine. From there, treatment is straightforward: Avoid eating your trigger food at least four hours before exercising. Unfortunately, this is a condition you're unlikely to outgrow.

tahini, and falafel), and even some cosmetic products, soaps, and hair care products. Because sesame seeds can produce severe reactions, read food labels carefully if you have this allergy.

A Closer Look at Delayed Food Allergies

IgE isn't the only bad boy when it comes to food allergies. A second category of food allergies, called delayed-type food allergies, is caused by cells in your body, which is why these allergies are also called cell-mediated food allergies. This category includes several specific diseases, and while they're not as common as immediate food allergies—they affect roughly five to ten out of every ten thousand people—they can still pose serious problems.

With this type of allergy, like all food allergies, certain cells of your immune system respond to a food protein. When you ingest that food protein, your immune system triggers those cells to react. Although any food can cause delayed food allergies, the most common triggers are allergens from milk, soy, wheat, egg, beef, corn, rice, fish, shellfish, and nuts. Just as with immediate food allergies, you could also be allergic to more than one of these foods.

Unlike immediate food allergies, though, delayed food allergies involve primarily one body system, the gastrointestinal tract. Because reactions happen slowly and are chronic in nature, symptoms aren't often closely related with ingesting the offending food.

The main symptoms for older children and adults include difficulty swallowing, abdominal pain, food impaction, vomiting, heartburn, and diarrhea. Younger children, however, often experience symptoms of gastro-esophageal reflux disease (like feeding difficulties and irritability), vomiting, bloody stools, and poor growth. Fortunately, symptoms from delayed food allergies are much less dangerous than immediate food allergies, since they don't carry the risk for anaphylaxis.

Yet don't think IgE is completely off the hook when it comes to delayed food allergies. IgE may play a role in one type of delayed food allergy called eosinophilic esophagitis (EoE), which we'll discuss below. Many individuals with EoE test positive for food-specific IgE, but at this point we're not entirely sure what role, if any, IgE may play in this allergy.

Among delayed food allergies, there are four specific diagnoses we'd like to highlight. Each has its own unique features and corresponding set of challenges.

Eosinophilic Esophagitis

This one's a mouthful, which is why we often refer to it as EoE. This disease involves the esophagus, which becomes inflamed mainly with a type of white blood cell called eosinophils that's common in other forms of chronic allergy disease (like asthma). Simply put, when you eat a food you're allergic to, the eosinophils respond.

As a result of this inflammation, you could experience symptoms of gastroesophageal reflux disease, like vomiting, regurgitation, abdominal or chest pain or heartburn, and even difficulty swallowing. In rare cases, you might suffer what's called food impaction, where food literally gets stuck in your esophagus, which could require emergency removal, as was the case with Jonathan, whom you met earlier.

Current estimates indicate that about one in ten thousand people suffer from EoE, and although it seems to be more common in children, adults can develop this disease as well. (In fact, it was first described in adults.) It affects more men than women and sticks around for life.

Eosinophilic Gastrointestinal Disease (EGID)

Eosinophils are also at work in this condition, better known as EGID, which also seems to mainly affect children. Yet rather than hanging out solely in the esophagus, as they do with EoE, these travel-happy white blood cells also invade parts or all of the gastrointestinal tract.

For some, when an offending food is eaten, inflammation with eosinophils can cause a wide variety of symptoms, including vomiting, swallowing problems, abdominal pain, diarrhea, food impaction, and slow growth. Yet not everyone who has eosinophils in their gastrointestinal tract has EGID, and not all EGID is caused by food allergy. Your doctor will need to make sure there's not another explanation for having this type of inflammation, like inflammatory bowel disease, for instance.

Fortunately, this form of eosinophilic disease is less common than EoE, but, like EoE, we currently believe it's a condition you'll probably have for life.

Allergic Colitis

Remember our little friend Claire, whom you met at the beginning of this chapter? Her mom suspected something was wrong when she saw blood in Claire's stool, which is a telltale sign of allergic colitis.

This condition is common in children under the age of one, who are usually healthy and growing well.

For some reason, they develop a delayed food allergy to milk or soy or, in some cases with breast-fed infants, some other food protein in the mother's diet. Symptoms can take days or weeks to appear and will also take time to resolve after the food allergen has been removed.

Fortunately, this is usually an easy condition to manage, since you simply take your child off milk or soy. For formula-fed infants, you may switch to a hypoallergenic formula. Or if your child's being breast-fed, the mother may have to cut some foods from her diet. Occasionally, it may be appropriate to consider weaning an infant to formula if the mother has to restrict her diet extensively, but we try to avoid that when possible.

By the time most children turn one, they've outgrown this allergy, and you can reintroduce milk or soy back into their diet.

Food-Protein-Induced Enterocolitis Syndrome

Try saying the name of this delayed food allergy several times in a row, and you'll understand why we call it FPIES (pronounced eff-pies). This strange-sounding condition can be scary for parents and children, and although it can cause severe reactions, most children recover well from it.

FPIES, which typically affects infants who don't have any other allergy, is a rare, cell-driven immune response in the gastrointestinal system to one or more specific foods. Milk, soy, rice, and other grains are the most common triggers. It often shows up in children who have early feeding trouble, usually with formula, or children who have recently been introduced to solid foods like infant cereals or formula, many of which are made with dairy or soy. Some children don't need to eat a large quantity of their offending food, since trace amounts can trigger a reaction.

While poor growth can be a red flag in some children, diarrhea and vomiting, sometimes severe, are the main symptoms. These symptoms usually begin about two hours after eating the trigger food, although the timing of reactions can vary by an hour or so on either side. While some symptoms like runny stools are mild, they can also be life-threatening, because some children can go into shock. This happens when the vomiting and diarrhea become so severe that the child experiences severe dehydration.

Warning signs of shock include weakness; dizziness; fainting; skin that looks pale and feels clammy and cool; a weak, fast pulse; shallow, fast breathing; extreme thirst; and confusion or anxiety. If you suspect your child has FPIES and they have a reaction with recurrent vomiting and/or diarrhea, seek medical attention. At that point, your child will be treated with intravenous fluids. Although you might wonder if you should use an epinephrine injector when you first see signs of shock as you would for immediate food allergies, there's no evidence that epinephrine is beneficial for FPIES.

Ironically, most parents learn about this condition when their child has such a severe reaction that they're rushed to the hospital or emergency room. Unfortunately, it's a tricky condition to diagnose—the only way to confirm it is through a food challenge—which is why you should work with an allergist to determine if your child might have this condition. Your doctor will also help you determine how to handle this condition, especially in emergency situations. In some cases, mild reactions can be treated at home with an oral electrolyte rehydration like Pedialyte, for instance.

Fortunately, children usually outgrow FPIES by the time they're four or five. Until then, avoiding the offending food is the best way to prevent reactions.

chapter 7

The Doctor Will See You Now

If you suspect you have a food allergy, you're probably a little on edge these days—and for good reason. You think food has become your foe, and you're no longer sure what you can or can't eat. It's like you're walking through a landmine every time you put food in your mouth, and for some people that anxiety can often be as troubling as the physical symptoms of a reaction.

That's why getting an accurate diagnosis is so important. Of course, with the rising cost of health care, it's tempting to play doctor and call your own shots. Yet while you might get away with self-diagnosing some food intolerances, you can't do that with food allergies. Food allergies are more serious than food intolerances, and if you diagnose yourself with the wrong food allergy—for instance, maybe you think you're allergic to fish when you're really allergic to shellfish—you could jeopardize your health.

On the flip side, you could diagnose yourself with a food allergy when, in reality, you have no allergy to food. Remember, after all, in chapter 3 when we told you about a study in which over 30 percent of people believed they had a food allergy when the real numbers hover closer to 4 percent of children and about 2 percent of adults? This may be less dangerous but no less debilitating as diagnosing yourself with the wrong allergy.

No doubt you'll have cut certain foods from your diet, which could lead to nutritional deficiencies. Following an avoidance diet can also be socially isolating, especially for kids who are often not allowed to go to parties or eat school lunches with their friends and may even be bullied more than kids without food allergies, according to a recent study. Living with a food allergy is tough enough for people who have been accurately diagnosed. Why would you want to go through that if you don't have to?

So if you do think you have a food allergy, whom should you see first—your family physician or an allergist? What tests can you expect, and how do you treat food allergies? We'll address all of those questions—and more—in this chapter.

Whom Should You Call for Help?

When you get sick, whom do you call? (And, no, your mom doesn't count!) If you said your family physician, that's not a bad place to start if you suspect you have a food allergy. A general physician may not be able to diagnose or treat your food allergy, but he or she can evaluate your symptoms and send you to the appropriate expert. Note that many insurance companies require a referral to see a specialist, which is why it's wise to start with a generalist like an internist, pediatrician, or family practitioner.

If your symptoms include hives, rashes, lip swelling, coughing, or shortness of breath soon after eating something, all of which point to an immediate food allergy, you should see an allergist. However, if you have abdominal pain, vomiting, nausea, gastroesophageal reflux disease, difficulty swallowing, choking, gagging, or food getting stuck in your throat, it makes sense to pay a visit to a gastroenterologist.

Itchy Mouth, Hives, Rashes—
Diagnosing Immediate Food Allergies

Diagnosing an immediate food allergy is often straightforward, but it can be a little tricky. Fortunately, though, allergists have a number of diagnostic tools at their disposal.

For starters, your medical history will play a large role in your diagnosis, which is why it's helpful to write down what you can remember about any suspicious foods or meals, especially if there were lots of ingredients. (If you're keeping a food diary as we suggested in chapter 1, bring that with you.) Be prepared to answer a lot of questions about your reactions to food. The allergist will also ask you about other allergies or allergy-related diseases and do a physical exam, checking for signs of allergic diseases.

From there, your allergist will determine which tests you might need. They could include any—or all—of the tests listed below.

Skin test

In this test, which is often the first one most people undergo, your skin will be scratched or pricked with an extract of the food you suspect you're allergic to. If you have IgE antibody to that food, you'll develop a bump that looks like a mosquito bite within minutes, indicating that histamine has been released as a result of specific IgE-triggering mast cells. Your skin will usually swell, too.

If you have no reaction, you can be pretty sure you don't have an immediate allergy to that food. However, if you do have a reaction, that doesn't necessarily mean you're allergic to the food. In some situations, you might have a small amount of IgE antibody to that food but not be truly allergic to the food, meaning that you can eat the food without any issues. You might also be cross-reacting to a protein in that food that's similar to a protein in another food or even an environmental allergen like pollen. This is why it's crucial to work with an allergist, who can interpret your results.

Because this test can be so sensitive, it may not be used if you've had a history of particularly severe reactions to food. Also, certain medications like antihistamines interfere with results, so you'll have to stop those medications before undergoing this test.

Blood test

This test can be a good option for people who have severe reactions to food allergies, people who can't go off their medication to undergo skin testing, and people who have certain skin conditions like severe and extensive eczema. It's also often used repeatedly over time to get a better sense of whether you may have outgrown your food allergy.

Like the skin test, a blood test goes on the hunt for IgE. A small amount of your blood will be drawn and sent to a lab.

If no allergen-specific IgE is found, you probably don't have an immediate allergy to that food, although there are sometimes false negatives. If, however, the test does find IgE, that still doesn't guarantee that you have a food allergy. However, the higher the IgE in your blood, the more likely it is that you do have a food allergy.

Surprisingly, your family physician can oversee this test. Yet because this test is poorly predictive by itself, misinterpretation of the test leads to many false positives. That's why you should have this test performed by an allergist, who can correctly interpret the results.

Food challenge

This is the gold standard of testing for immediate food allergies, and it's often performed if the medical history, skin test, and blood test don't show conclusive results. Allergists also use it to determine if you've outgrown an allergy.

As the name implies, this test challenges your body to respond to a suspect food. Although there are various ways to administer this test—in some cases, you may know what you're eating, while in other cases, you won't—the premise is the same: You'll be asked to eat the suspect food while your allergist watches for a reaction. If you do have a reaction, you're almost certainly allergic to that food.

Because this test carries a risk of serious reactions, you should never try this at home. Only do this in the presence of your allergist, who's trained to give emergency treatment if necessary.

Treating Immediate Food Allergies

So what do you do if you're diagnosed with an immediate food allergy? Unfortunately, there's currently only one treatment option: Go on an elimination diet, where you completely avoid the food. You may only have to follow this diet until you've outgrown the allergy, but in situations where outgrowing a food allergy is unlikely, you'll have to follow this diet for life.

You should also consider wearing a medical alert bracelet, especially if you've had a severe allergic reaction in the past. In case you ever lose consciousness, this bracelet could save your life. Make sure your bracelet includes your known allergies and the name and phone number of an emergency contact.

When Your Gut Gets Involved— Diagnosing Delayed Food Allergies

Delayed food allergies are different from immediate food allergies so it makes sense that they are diagnosed differently. Yet when you first see your gastroenterologist about a suspected delayed food allergy, you'll still be asked about your medical history and will undergo a physical exam.

Your doctor will then run you through one or all of the tests below.

Blood test

Blood will often be tested for two things: IgE and eosinophils, which, as you may remember from the previous chapter, are white blood cells associated with inflammation in some delayed food allergy reactions. IgE, of course, primarily suggests an immediate food allergy, which the doctor is trying to rule out. (Some people, though, do have both immediate and delayed food allergies. Remember, too, that specific IgE is often found in some delayed food allergies like EoE.) Eosinophils, on the other hand, could indicate inflammation in the body.

Nutritional evaluation

Because gastrointestinal problems with delayed food allergies often cause food not to be absorbed as well, you may be screened for vitamin D, iron, and protein deficiencies. If your vitamin D blood level is below thirty-two nanograms per milliliter, your doctor will recommend taking vitamin D supplements. Likewise, if you test low for iron or proteins, you'll be advised to supplement your diet.

Antacid medication

Many individuals who are diagnosed with EoE complain of acid reflux symptoms like heartburn and vomiting. Because it's unclear at this point whether you have acid reflux or a delayed food allergy, your doctor will most likely recommend taking an antacid medication for six weeks. If your symptoms disappear after six weeks, you probably have acid reflux, and no further testing will be required. If, though, the symptoms haven't resolved, your doctor will run additional tests for delayed food allergies, and you'll continue the medication until you determine which food is bothering you.

Endoscopy

An endoscopy is the gold standard by which doctors diagnose delayed food allergies. During this test, the gastroenterologist will examine your esophagus, stomach, and small bowel using a thin, flexible tube. The procedure takes only about ten minutes, but ultimately, it will allow your doctor to see if you have any inflammation in your gastrointestinal tract. If so, you probably have a delayed food allergy.

Patch testing

Patch testing is sometimes used to help identify relevant food allergens. In this test, you'll wear a small patch that's been exposed to the food protein you're suspected to be allergic to. If you have a reaction, usually a small area that looks like poison ivy, after wearing the patch for three days, you may be allergic to that food.

Elimination diet

For delayed food allergies, testing often doesn't accurately identify the trigger foods. As a result, your doctor may recommend following an elimination diet for six weeks, where you avoid one food or a set of foods believed to be the problem. After the six week period, you'll undergo another endoscopy to see if the inflammation has diminished. If the inflammation hasn't diminished, your doctor may add more foods to your elimination diet, which you'll follow for another six weeks. You'll then undergo another endoscopy, and the process will continue. How long could this go on? That's up to you and your doctor. You may also need to discuss other treatment options or reevaluate the diagnosis.

One point we should mention: You might undergo all of this testing and still not have a definitive answer. Fortunately, this doesn't happen frequently, but we do want you to be aware of this possibility and know that modern medicine does have its limits.

Finding Relief from Delayed Food Allergies

No matter what type of delayed food allergy you're diagnosed with, dietary changes are the recommended treatment. To prevent symptoms, you have to avoid eating the food you're allergic to.

What if you do eat your offending food? Fortunately,

you don't have to worry about experiencing a life-threatening reaction like anaphylaxis. However, regularly eating this food could damage your esophagus. In some individuals, the esophagus can narrow to the point that swallowing is difficult, if not impossible.

While dietary changes are the main treatment, you can also take swallowed steroid inhalers, especially if you're not ready to change your eating habits. Maybe you're going through a stressful situation in your family or work life or you're traveling to a different country for several weeks and can't guarantee that you can avoid your trigger food.

Note, though, that swallowed steroid inhalers are only a Band-Aid treatment. They provide short-term relief but aren't ideal for the long haul, since they often cause side effects like candida, a fungal infection of the esophagus that could cause suppressed growth in children; osteoporosis; and hypertension. We try to avoid recommending their use for longer than three months, especially in children. That being said, though, for some individuals, long-term treatment might be the best option at this time, since other medications, like montelukast and cromolyn, which have been used for IgE-mediated allergies and have been studied in treating delayed allergies, have not been shown to be effective.

You'll also need to see your gastroenterologist—and your allergist if you have immediate food allergies, too—at least every year, if not more regularly, for the rest of your life. (So make sure you choose a doctor you like!) During those exams, your doctor will check that your dietary changes are keeping inflammation at bay and giving you the nourishment you need.

A Word About Alternative Treatments

Alternative medicine is hot these days: Roughly 38 percent of adults use some type of complementary and alternative medicine to achieve health and well-being, according to the National Center for Complementary and Alternative Medicine. Among those therapies are procedures to diagnose and treat food allergies, but do they work?

That's a question many of our patients ask. In fact, some of our patients have tried these alternative forms of treatment. In many cases, they've completed many of the tests we've already discussed, but because we still can't pinpoint their problem, they go searching for answers in other places. In other situations, people are leery of modern medicine and simply prefer alternative forms of medicine. Or it may be that these are health-savvy individuals who are interested in doing a more thorough investigation of their condition.

Before we give you our take, let's look at some of the most common alternative therapies that allegedly diagnose your food allergy:

Cytotoxic testing: After being exposed to specific allergens, your blood cells undergo microscopic evaluation. Changes in the cells supposedly suggest an allergic reaction.

Provocation-neutralization test: Increasing amounts of your trigger food are injected into your skin until a wheal, a mosquito-like bump that indicates allergy, appears. The dose is then decreased until the wheal disappears.

Electrodermal testing: This test detects energy imbalances in your body by using a galvanometer, an instrument that indicates the presence or strength of a small electric current. If you have an energy imbalance, it's assumed you have a food allergy.

Applied kinesiology: You hold the food you think you're allergic to while your muscle strength is tested. The practitioner applies counterpressure to your outstretched arm. Because the theory goes that nutritional deficiencies result in muscle weakness, you're apparently allergic to that food if you're unable to resist that pressure.

Pulse test: Your pulse is taken before and after eating certain foods. A higher pulse supposedly indicates you're allergic to that food.

Serum IgG: This test measures IgG antibodies to certain foods. Practitioners claim that high IgG antibody readings indicate an allergy to that specific food.

ELISA/ACT test: Your lymphocytes, or white blood cells, are tested against dozens of foods to see how they respond.

Here are three alternative remedies that claim to treat your allergy:

Acupuncture: This ancient Chinese medicine is founded on the belief that every individual has a flow of qi, or life energy, and when qi is blocked, your health suffers. Yet by opening up the meridians, or the pathways through which qi flows through the body, your body can heal itself of various conditions, including food allergies.

Homeopathy: Homeopathy claims to stimulate the body's natural defenses against food allergies and help the body respond less to allergens, mainly through the use of remedies made from natural substances.

Supplements: Through a variety of vitamins, amino acids, and enzymes, your body is brought back into chemical balance to help you overcome your food allergy.

Now back to our original question: Do any of these work? In a word, no. We do have an open mind, though, as we know it's possible that future procedures to diagnose and test for food allergies may come from outside conventional medicine. Yet there's currently no research to support any of these therapies, and, because of that, we can't endorse them.

While people do claim to get better after having undergone some of these therapies, the evidence right now is purely anecdotal. Unlike the procedures we use to diagnose and test for food allergies, which have been subjected to clinical studies, these therapies are unproven.

If, though, you're still interested in trying one of these therapies, know that there are pitfalls, and you need to examine the risks carefully, especially if you have an immediate food allergy. Many of these therapies place you in direct contact with your allergen, and with anaphylaxis a possibility for people with immediate food allergies, this could put you in danger. And because these are unproven tests, there's no guarantee that any results you get will be accurate. Plus, you'll usually have to foot the bill, since insurance doesn't typically cover these therapies or tests. As a result, you could pay a pretty penny for some of these things without any guarantee you'll get the answers you're seeking.

Most important, if you decide to try an alternative therapy, continue to see your allergist or gastroenterologist. Your doctor can help ensure that the treatment isn't harmful to your health and check that you're not depriving yourself of the nutrients you need. If your child is undergoing these therapies, your doctor will make sure your child is still growing properly.

How Do You Know If You've Outgrown a Food Allergy?

You don't need science to figure out when you've outgrown your clothes, your shoes, even your taste in music. But what about a food allergy?

For immediate food allergies; your allergist will determine when it's time to retest you or your child. When the time is right, your allergist may recommend undergoing a blood test and possibly a food challenge to see if you've outgrown the allergy. If you pass the challenge, meaning that you have no reaction, you can safely re-introduce that food into your diet. In fact, we encourage individuals who have outgrown their food allergy to eat the food they were once allergic to on a regular basis. If, however, you react during a challenge, your allergist will probably recommend waiting another six to twelve months before testing again.

Because they don't carry risk of serious reactions, delayed food allergies are a little different. Most children outgrow some forms of delayed food allergies by the time they're toddlers, which is usually when your gastroenterologist will recommend reintroducing the trigger food back into the diet in small amounts. If you don't see a reaction, it's safe to assume your child has probably outgrown this allergy, and this food can gradually be added back to the diet. Unfortunately, conditions like eosinophilic esophagitis and other eosinophilic gastrointestinal diseases are rarely outgrown.

Ironically, you may find out your child has outgrown an allergy by accidental exposure. For instance, maybe your milk-allergic child accidentally eats a muffin that contains milk but doesn't react.

If this happens, inform your doctor, especially if your child has an immediate food allergy. While tolerating something like milk in a muffin might mean that your child is less sensitive to milk, you can't assume your child can now drink milk.

We know that a large percentage of children who remain milk-allergic can tolerate at least some milk as an ingredient in another food. But from an accidental-ingestion perspective, you can't be sure how much milk as an ingredient—or in what foods that contain milk—your child can tolerate. If your assumptions are incorrect, you could put your child at serious risk, which is why you should always consult your doctor first.

chapter 8

Living with Food Allergies

If only food allergies were like a bad date—just give them the brush-off and you wouldn't have to worry about them again. Unfortunately, though, food allergies are clingy little creatures and stick with you no matter where you go.

So if you can't shake your food allergy (remember, though, that some people will outgrow their food allergy), what can you do? The only choice you have: Learn to thrive despite it.

Of course, that may be easier said than done, especially in a world where food ingredients are often tough to decipher and UFOs, or unidentified food objects, are everywhere. Yet there is a bright side (and we know this from the hundreds of patients we've treated): The majority of individuals who have a food allergy have no trouble fitting into society. They learn what precautions they should take, they pay careful attention to their diet, and they rarely have issues with their food allergy. And when they do have problems, they know how to respond.

Want to be one of those individuals? In this chapter, we'll give you the tools you need to successfully manage your food allergy, whether you're at home, school, a restaurant, or on vacation. With this information in your toolbox, you can keep those allergies from being little more than a nuisance.

Dealing with an Allergic Reaction to Food

Even on the strictest of avoidance diets, accidents happen, and you could unintentionally consume your trigger food. If that happens, you need to know how to respond, especially if you have an immediate food allergy. While delayed food allergies never involve anaphylaxis, all immediate food allergies have the potential to cause this severe reaction.

This doesn't mean that if you have an immediate food allergy, you'll experience anaphylaxis—researchers are currently looking at ways to determine who might be more at risk for anaphylaxis—but you should still consider yourself at risk and take appropriate precautions. Have an emergency plan in action, carry epinephrine with you wherever you go, and if the allergic individual is a child, make sure all of your child's caregivers are aware of this plan. To help ease your fears, though, remember that reactions from food allergies rarely lead to hospital admission or death.

How you respond to an immediate food allergy reaction will depend on your symptoms. Follow these guidelines:

If you have mild symptoms: these include itchy mouth, a few hives around the mouth or face, mild itch, or mild nausea or discomfort

Do this: Take an antihistamine like Benadryl. If your symptoms progress, administer epinephrine.

If you have more severe symptoms: symptoms that involve one or more of the following—shortness of breath, wheezing, repetitive coughing, paleness, blueness, faint feeling, weak pulse, dizziness, confusion, tight or hoarse throat, trouble breathing or swallowing, obstructive swelling in the tongue and/or lips, many hives over the body—or symptoms that involve a combination from different body areas (e.g., hives, itchy rashes, or swelling and vomiting or crampy pain)

>   *Do this:* Give epinephrine immediately and call
>   911. If you have asthma, you can take your med-
>   ication with epinephrine, but don't ever use your
>   medication in place of epinephrine. Asthma medi-
>   cation can't reverse the symptoms of anaphylaxis.

What about reactions to delayed food allergies? Be-cause these aren't life-threatening, the best response is just to give your symptoms some time to ease. You can also use a few over-the-counter medications to treat common symptoms.

If, for instance, you're having reflux symptoms or heartburn, take an antacid medication. Feeling a little gassy? Take a product with simethicone (like Gas-X). Or if you have abdominal pain, you can pop acetamin-ophen (like Tylenol).

If, however, you have prolonged abdominal pain, diarrhea, or constipation, probiotic supplements may sometimes help, since they may reduce pain and regu-late bowel movements. Just make sure you read the label ingredients on these supplements, which can contain surprising ingredients like lactose that you may not be able to tolerate.

The Skinny on Epinephrine

Epinephrine is the most potent medication against anaphylaxis, since it reverses the symptoms and helps prevent them from progressing. It's available by prescription only in self-injectable devices like EpiPen and Twinject. Your doctor will show you how to use it, but you can also find video demonstrations online at www.epipen.com/how-to-use-epipen or www.twinject.com.

To help you use epinephrine more effectively, follow these tips:

- Make sure you get the right dose. Autoinjectors come in two dosing strengths, one for young children and another for individuals who weigh sixty-six pounds or more. In some cases, even if you're at a lower weight, your physician may decide to move you up to the adult-dose epinephrine.
- Carry two doses of epinephrine with you wherever you go, especially if you have a history of severe allergic reactions. In some cases, you may need two doses during an allergic reaction, especially if you make a mistake trying to administer the first.

(continued)

- Pay attention to the expiration date. The drug becomes less effective after it's expired.
- Store epinephrine at room temperature, and never leave it in the car, because it could get too hot or too cold.
- Let family and friends know where you store your epinephrine in the house and always carry it on you when you're out.
- If your school-aged child has the allergy, talk with school personnel about their regulations for carrying epinephrine self-injectors, and make sure your child or key personnel at the school have immediate access to this medication.

Dealing with Anxieties About Food Allergies

Many of our patients have expressed anxiety about their food allergies. They've gotten so worked up at times that they've become terrified of eating.

Anxiety also strikes parents of food-allergic children. One of Dr. Wayne's patients, for instance, is an eight-year-old girl who's outgrown many of her allergies, but because the mother is so petrified that her daughter will have a reaction, she won't allow her daughter to attend school. Instead, the mother has chosen to homeschool her child.

It's certainly understandable that you may be anxious about your allergy or your child's allergy, but let us put four of your most common fears to rest.

Fear #1: I'm Not Going to Be Able to Live a Normal Life

We say: With the help of a qualified medical professional, food allergies can be successfully managed so that you can do everything you would (with the exception of eating your trigger food) if you didn't have a food allergy. Go to school? Eat out with friends? Take a vacation? Even with a food allergy, you can do all of those things—and then some. You'll just need to plan more carefully than others.

Fear #2: I'm Worried That I'm Going to React from Simply Being Near the Food I'm Allergic To

We say: Dangerous reactions are most commonly caused by accidental ingestion of foods, not casual exposure. Although it's true that if the particles of the food get airborne severe reactions can occur, studies have found that skin exposure or being exposed to molecules that cause food to smell don't pose a serious threat to food-allergic individuals.

Fear #3: I'm Scared That I'm Going to Have an Anaphylactic Reaction, Even Wind Up in the Hospital

We say: While everybody who has an immediate food allergy should be prepared to treat an anaphylactic reaction, the percentage of people who actually experience this severe reaction is low. If you do have a severe reaction, epinephrine is very safe and effective.

If you're still feeling on edge and your anxiety has begun to interrupt your daily life, consider talking with a psychologist. We actually have a psychologist on our team who specializes in helping people deal with fears like these, so if you're having difficulty coping, reach out to a qualified professional.

Learning How to Read Labels

If you've revamped your diet in an effort to eat healthier, you're no doubt already familiar with food labels.

They're packed with information about calories, protein, fats, sugar, and sodium levels. Yet if you've been diagnosed with a food allergy, food labels will become your best friend, too.

That's because food labels also list every ingredient used to make that particular food, thanks in large part to a labeling law called the Food Allergen Labeling and Consumer Protection Act (FALCPA). As a result, you'll be able to see whether a food contains common allergens like nuts, milk, and eggs. Just be aware, though, that these allergens can hide in ingredients you may not be familiar with.

If you're not sure whether a food contains a particular allergen, especially if you have a less common food allergy, call the manufacturer and ask. Also, remember that manufacturers often change their recipes, which is why you should never assume that a food you've eaten for years is safe. You still need to check labels to make sure nothing's changed.

No matter, follow this rule for all foods: When in doubt, leave it out (of your grocery cart, that is).

Decoding Food Labels

There's a reason food labels contain certain allergy warnings: In 2004, Congress passed the Food Allergen Labeling and Consumer Protection Act (FALCPA), requiring manufacturers to identify ingredients from eight major food allergens, including milk, egg, soybean, wheat, peanut, tree nut (identifying the specific tree nut), fish (identifying the specific fish species), and crustacean (identifying the specific species—however, FALCPA doesn't recognize mollusks, like scallops, oysters, and clams as major allergens).

It doesn't matter how much of the allergen is used—any amount requires the manufacturer to list it in food products. According to FALCPA, allergens have to be listed in one of three ways:

1) In the ingredient list (i.e., the list might read "wheat," "soy," or "milk")
2) In parentheses following the derivative of the food protein—i.e., "casein (milk)"
3) Below the ingredient list in a "contains" statement (i.e., "contains wheat and soy")

Note, though, that advisory statements like "may contain [certain allergen]" or "produced in a facility that also processes [certain allergen]" are voluntary.

How worried should you be about these advisory statements? That may depend on your allergy. For example, the risk associated with cross-contamination is somewhat different for an allergy like milk than it is for peanuts. Here's why:

When there's a trace contamination of milk because of shared equipment, the contamination will be spread evenly through the next batch. So the individual risk of each bite for people with an immediate food allergy to milk is negligible.

However, if you have eosinophilic esophagitis and you're allergic to milk, you should avoid foods that carry these advisory warnings. If you eat these foods regularly, you could possibly get a consistent dose of milk in your diet, which could be enough to cause inflammation.

Meanwhile, for peanuts (or tree nuts), the nature of the contamination may be a small piece in one bite that's enough to provoke a reaction. So even though the individual risk of each bite is low, if you get the wrong bite and eat that fragment, it could be enough to cause a serious reaction. That's why we generally recommend paying close attention to these advisory labels if you have a peanut or tree nut allergy.

Individuals also vary in terms of how sensitive they are to small amounts of exposure, and some probably don't

(continued)

need to worry as much about precautionary labels. Unfortunately, we currently don't have the means of identifying who is at greatest risk, and because the nature of cross-contamination is likely to be intermittent, a history of always tolerating products with warning labels can't be taken as strong evidence that it's okay for you to continue eating these products. Bottom line: Heed these warnings.

Coping with Food Allergies in the Home

Dealing with a food allergy at home seems easy. After all, you control what comes into your house, right? That might be true if you're living alone. However, if you have several family members living under one roof and only one of you has a food allergy, you'll have to decide whether or not you bring the offending food into the house.

That's something only you and your family can decide. In fact, we don't like to dictate what families should do, since each situation is unique and needs to be judged differently. We have many patients who have a food-allergic child yet allow the allergen in the house. Other families, however, have decided this isn't right for them and have banned all risky foods from the house.

To help you make this decision, answer these questions:

- What type of food allergy does your family member have—immediate or delayed?
- How old are your family members? How responsible are they?
- How difficult will it be to eliminate this food from your family's diet?
- How will eliminating this food change the quality of your family members' lives?
- Is your family good about cleaning up after meals? Or is the kitchen often left a mess after meals or snacks?
- Does the allergic individual have a history of severe reactions or reactions provoked by small exposures?

If you decide to allow the allergen in your house, make sure you clean plates, utensils, and cookware thoroughly. Otherwise, cross-contamination could occur. Fortunately, though, there's a relation between the amount of exposure and the likelihood and severity of reactions, meaning that how much you eat will determine whether you have a reaction and how severe that reaction will be. The good news is that most reactions from cross-contamination aren't likely to be severe.

Overall, remember that most serious accidental reactions are the results of unintentionally eating something with the allergen in it. So focus your attention on strategies to minimize that risk.

To do that, make these strategies part of your everyday habits:

- Wash pots, pans, cutting boards, and utensils with soap and water before cooking. Wash them again between preparations for safe (allergy-free) and unsafe (allergen-containing) foods. You might also consider buying separate cutting boards for safe and unsafe foods.

- Cook allergen-free foods first, especially if you're cooking unsafe foods at the same time. Then cover the safe food and keep it away from unsafe foods, especially any that are prone to spattering.

- Watch out for airborne exposure. Some foods like flour are easily airborne, and in those cases, care should be given to prevent exposure to an allergic family member. The rule of thumb here is that it's not the smell of a food—the molecules you smell aren't the proteins and, therefore, don't trigger reactions—but airborne particles that can be a problem. For instance, somebody making a peanut butter sandwich in the same room isn't a problem, but actively shelling peanuts nearby could be. If you do find yourself in that situation, leave the room.

- Whenever you handle unsafe foods, wash your hands, especially right before you serve meals.
- Keep utensils for safe foods separate from unsafe foods. Also, never serve allergen-free foods with the same utensil that's used to serve unsafe foods.
- During cleanup, wash all surfaces, including cutting boards, kitchen counters, and tables, with soap and water. Use something other than a sponge, where allergens often get stuck. Good alternatives include a disposable towel or a cloth that can be washed.
- Store all foods in sealed containers. This prevents them from splattering in the fridge and causing accidental contamination.
- When grilling, which can pose significant risks for cross-contamination, place foil on the grill whenever you cook, prepare safe foods away from unsafe foods, and give the grill a thorough cleaning after each use.

As mentioned above, while cross-contamination is certainly a concern, there's an even bigger risk that can happen when allergens are allowed in the house: Your food-allergic family member could accidentally eat the wrong food. For instance, maybe you have a child who's allergic to milk, but instead of drinking his cup of soy milk, he picks up his brother's cup of cow's milk. These types of mistakes are more worrisome, since they're more likely to cause severe reactions.

That's why it's crucial to devise a plan to avoid these mistakes. Some ideas: Assign your food-allergic child a certain colored cup, use color-coded labels to distinguish between safe and unsafe foods. And be vigilant about food being left around the house, again, much of the risk also depends on the age of the allergic household member.

Simple Substitutions for At-Home Cooking

Don't think that if you have a food allergy, you have to exist on a bland, tasteless diet. With all of the products on the market these days, you can easily find something to fit your needs.

Our advice? Scour your grocery story to unearth these products. But read those labels: Some of these substitutes can contain the allergen you're allergic to. For instance, commercial egg substitutes can contain egg whites, while some products that are labeled dairy-free, like nondairy creamers, may actually contain milk.

You can also use easy substitutes when cooking at home. Follow these tips to make allergy-free swaps:

For one egg, use these substitutes:

- 1 teaspoon baking power, 1 tablespoon water, 1 tablespoon vinegar
- 1 teaspoon yeast dissolved in 1/4 cup warm water
- 1 1/2 tablespoons water, 1 1/2 tablespoons oil, 1 teaspoon baking powder
- 1 package gelatin, 2 tablespoons warm water (but don't mix until you're ready to use)

For one cup of wheat flour, use these substitutes:

- 7/8 cup rice flour
- 5/8 cup potato-starch flour
- 1 cup soy flour plus 1/4 cup potato-starch flour
- 1 cup corn flour

For one cup of milk, use these substitutes:

- 1 cup water, fruit juice, soy milk, or rice milk

Sending Your Food-Allergic Child
to School

School can be a scary experience for kids, even if they
don't have a food allergy. But if you have a child with
a food allergy, it can be equally scary since you may
worry about sending your child away from your protective wing.

These worries prompt some parents, including the
one we mentioned earlier, to homeschool their children. Yet we don't believe a food allergy a reason for
homeschooling. At the very least, your child's food allergy should be at the bottom of the list when deciding
whether to homeschool.

There are also many allergy-free schools, but, to be
honest, we're not fans of these schools, since it's easy to
let down your guard and get lulled into a false sense of
security. The school can also get lulled into that false
sense of security, thinking that it has all allergens covered, when in fact it is directing most of its efforts to-
ward only one allergen.

The good news, though, is that schools have gotten
better about dealing with food allergies. In fact, 83 percent of parents reported that their child's daycare or
preschool provided at least one accommodation for children with food allergies (e.g., banning treats or foods

brought in from home, creating separate eating areas for food-allergic children, or posting food allergy plans) while 79 percent of parents reported that their child's elementary school offered these types of accommodations, according to the "C. S. Mott Children's Hospital National Poll on Children's Health."

To keep your child safe, here are four strategies you can follow:

Inform the school about your child's allergy and create an action plan: Let the school know exactly what your child's allergy is and how to handle a reaction. In fact, you should give the school an action plan you've created with your child's allergist in case an emergency does arise. If you have older children, particularly those in high school, think about what might happen if your child has a reaction not only during the school day but also after school, when your child may be participating in extracurricular activities off school grounds. For help with all of this, check out the "Back-to School Tool Kit from the Food Allergy and Anaphylaxis Network" (www.foodallergy .org/section/back-to-school-tool-kit). The kit has been designed for all grade levels and includes information that teachers, school staff, doctors, and other children should know about your child's allergy.

Ask about the school's food policies: Does the school allow food in the classroom or is food allowed only in the cafeteria? Can kids bring in treats on special occasions like birthdays or holidays? If so, how is that food managed? Once you learn this, you can help tailor guidelines to minimize your child's risk of exposure. Just don't ask all of the other parents to cater to your child's food allergy, since that can create unwanted backlash. Besides, delegating this responsibility to anybody else is unwise. People who aren't used to dealing with food allergies can get confused about what is safe and what's not safe and forget that they may be using something that's not appropriate for somebody with a particular allergy. Do you really want to take that risk?

Decide who will handle the epinephrine: If your child has an immediate food allergy, epinephrine must be available in case a reaction does occur. If your child is young, determine who will be responsible for the epinephrine. Is there a school nurse? If not, what role will the teacher play? Even more important, where will the epinephrine be kept? Once your child turns twelve or thirteen years old, he or she should be able to carry their own epinephrine.

Educate your child: Make sure you're doing all that you can to educate your child about his or her particular allergy. That includes teaching your child from a young age how to minimize risk of exposure, including reading food labels and not accepting food from other children. This is important for children with immediate food allergies, but even children with delayed food allergies need to be reminded of the dangers of eating foods they're allergic to. Many of Dr. Qian's school-aged patients have strayed from their diets at school, only to wind up with recurring problems.

Dining Out with Your Food Allergy

Going out to eat can be troublesome for people with food allergies. Unlike cooking at home, where you can control what you're eating, you have to place great faith in the kitchen staff when you eat out, and that can be a tremendous obstacle to overcome.

Yet you don't have to avoid restaurants completely. Instead, employ some allergy smarts and learn how to spot risky situations to minimize the chance of a reaction, especially if you have an immediate food allergy.

Follow these five strategies to minimize your risk:

Choose allergy-friendly restaurants whenever possible:
The increasing awareness of allergies has prompted numerous restaurants, especially chains, to create special menus for allergic individuals. For instance, T.G.I. Friday's, Ruby Tuesday, Baskin-Robbins, Culver's, and Qdoba publish information about allergens in their foods. Chains, by the way, tend to be more reliable in handling allergies than mom-and-pop shops. However, some local businesses cater specifically to individuals with food allergies and other restrictions. Likewise, higher-end restaurants also generally handle food allergies better than other restaurants. If you're not sure, call the restaurant or view their Web site online. There are also Web sites like Allergy Eats! (www.allergyeats.com) and AllerDine (www.allerdine.com) that provide guides to allergy-friendly restaurants.

Be wary of high-risk restaurants: Although allergy-friendly restaurants seem to be on the rise, there are some non-allergy-friendly restaurants you should avoid. Buffets, bakeries, salad bars, and ice cream shops are especially risky for people with nut allergies. Restaurants that serve prepackaged foods can also be troublesome, depending on your allergy. It's quite possible that the person preparing the food won't have read the labels and won't know what allergens might be in the food. Then there are certain types of restaurants that are higher risk, depending on what your allergy is. For example, if you have a shellfish or fish allergy, going to a seafood joint like Long John Silver's or Red Lobster isn't wise. For people with fish allergies, ethnic restaurants like Chinese, Thai, and Vietnamese are also high-risk since many of their dishes use fish and fish ingredients, increasing the likelihood of cross-contamination. The same is true for many ethnic restaurants (i.e., Chinese, Indonesian, African, Thai, and Vietnamese) if you have a peanut or tree nut allergy, since nuts and nut products are used frequently in these cuisines. Ditto for those steak houses that serve free peanuts (and often let you throw them on the floor).

Chat with the waitstaff: When booking a reservation, tell the restaurant about your allergy and ask if the restaurant can accommodate your allergy. When you arrive at the restaurant, inform your server and ask specific questions about the menu, including what's in a particular food and how the food is prepared. If your server doesn't know, ask to speak to the manager or the chef. Yet even if the server does seem knowledgeable, be sure to ask that the chef be informed of your allergy. And by all means, if you don't trust what your server is telling you or your server isn't treating your allergy seriously, don't be afraid to leave. It's important, after all, that you trust the restaurant staff.

Carry a chef card: These cards help you communicate directly with the chef and kitchen staff about your allergy, since they ask you to list the foods you're allergic to and any related ingredients you can't eat. They also include a few tips on how to avoid cross-contamination. Carry them with you whenever you go out to eat and hand one to your server and request that it be passed to the chef. Print them on brightly colored paper so your card will stand out in the kitchen. (You can download a premade chef-card template through the Food Allergy and Anaphylaxis Network at www.foodallergy.org/files/media/chef-card1/chefcardtemplate.pdf.) Remember, too, that you'll need these if you're a mom who's breast-feeding a baby with a delayed food allergy. After all, if you eat the food your baby is allergic to, you'll pass it to your baby when breast-feeding, and that could kick off a bout of symptoms.

Watch out for sauces and desserts. Sauces and desserts might taste yummy, but they're also great hiding places for allergens. As a double whammy, desserts carry a high risk of cross-contamination, too. Order your foods sans sauce and either say no thank you to dessert (your waistline will thank you!) or, if you must, wait until you get home to eat an allergy-free dessert.

Taking Your Allergy on Vacation

When you take your next vacation, you'll need to make room for your food allergy—not physically of course, but in your planning. It's perfectly fine to travel with a food allergy, and as long as you take a few precautions—especially if you have an immediate food allergy—you and your food allergy can have a wonderful vacation.

Being an Allergy-Safe Road Warrior

For the majority of people with food allergies, traveling is no big deal. Yet because accidents can happen, there are some general guidelines we recommend to patients:

Get your medication in order: Several days before your trip, check that you have a good supply of epinephrine, especially if you're traveling to a remote area in another country. One of Dr. Wayne's patients, a college student, did a three-week backpacking trip through Asia, and, to manage his food allergy, we decided he should travel with extra EpiPens to be safe, although he never had to use one.

Wear a medical alert bracelet if you have an immediate food allergy or celiac disease: If you've read this book from the start (and kudos if you have), you'll remember that we recommended that if you fit these two categories, you should wear this bracelet all of the time, even at home. Yet it's even more important on the road, where anything can happen.

Avoid traveling alone, especially if you're going to remote areas: This holds true no matter what type of health condition you have, but if you have an immediate food allergy, don't take chances. Use the buddy system and make sure your buddy knows about your allergy and where you keep your epinephrine. You might also give your traveling companion a quick tutorial about how to use the epinephrine in case the need arises.

> *Be your own sleuth:* The Internet has made it easy to research your destination, so take advantage of it and do a little homework before you go. Check, for instance, restaurants that cater to people with food allergies or log on to an airline's Web site to check its allergy policies.

Welcome to the Friendly Skies

Flying poses a greater risk for people with immediate food allergies than delayed food allergies, as they have a risk of a severe reaction. Yet immediate food allergies are manageable with these tips:

> *Give advance warning:* When booking your flights, notify the airline that you or your child has a food allergy. There's a lot of variability in how airlines respond, but at least you've done your part in alerting them. You should also inform the flight attendants when you get on the plane, especially if you're allergic to peanuts, since more airlines are offering peanuts again. It might even be wise before you book your ticket to ask the airlines what snacks they serve on board. Check the airline's Web site, too, where many list their allergy policies.

Opt for early-morning flights whenever possible: You never know what the prior passengers in your seats were eating (or stuffed into the seat pocket in front of you), and early-morning flights give you greater assurance that the plane has been more thoroughly cleaned (which is often done at night), limiting the risk that you will run into your allergen.

Get a letter from your doctor stating why you need epinephrine: Without a letter, you may have trouble with airport security. The epinephrine might need to be in its original packaging, so check with the airline and FAA's policies before you travel. The Food and Allergy Anaphylaxis Network also recommends having the pharmacy's prescription label on your medication. Just don't pack the epinephrine in any checked baggage and expect to see it when you arrive at your destination. Airlines are notorious for losing luggage. Besides, you never know when you might need your medication.

BYOF: If you're flying during a meal, bring your own food. Most airlines do serve food on board, but because you can't always guarantee what's in those foods, it's best to take your own food on board.

Pit Stops: Eating on the Road

Remember the first time you ate at a restaurant in your hometown? No doubt you proceeded cautiously and alerted the chef and kitchen staff about your food allergy. Eating out on vacation should be no different from eating out at home. Follow the tips we outlined in the previous section and then pack these additional strategies in your suitcase:

Pack those chef cards: Continue to carry your chef cards with you, and if you're traveling to a foreign destination, get the cards in the local language, especially if you don't speak the language. (Although we can't vouch for the translations, we found a good site called Allergy Translation [www.allergytranslation.com] that offers these cards in over twenty-five different languages for a low price.) When you get to a restaurant, ask if anybody speaks English so you can convey your needs to that individual, who can then inform the chef. Yet if you ever feel uncomfortable or unsure about the food in a restaurant, leave. It's always better to be safe than sorry.

Go with what you know: If you're traveling in remote areas like the college student we mentioned above, stick with prepackaged, labeled food as much as possible. Choose major brand names, since they may be more diligent about issuing allergy warnings on their packages.

Consider taking a swallowed steroid inhaler if you have a delayed food allergy: If you have a delayed food allergy and think it's going to be difficult or downright impossible to avoid your trigger food, especially if you're traveling internationally, talk with your doctor about taking a swallowed steroid inhaler. Although individuals with delayed food allergies aren't at risk for anaphylaxis, they do have to worry about inflammation. By taking the steroid, you'll keep inflammation to a minimum in case you do eat your offending food. When you return home, you can gradually quit taking the steroids under the guidance of your doctor.

chapter 9

Will There Ever Be a Cure for Food Sensitivities?

Whether you have a food intolerance or a food allergy, you're probably wondering if you'll ever be able to eat food without having to worry about how your body will respond. Our answer? For some people, it may someday be possible.

When it comes to food allergies in particular, there's never been a better time to have hope. In recent years, researchers have made numerous advances in potential treatments.

Of course, curative treatments for food allergies don't exist right now. All we can tell you is how to avoid your allergen and relieve any symptoms you might experience from accidental ingestions. Yet studies have shown that some treatments for reducing sensitivity have been effective, and although these treatments aren't yet recommended for routine use, they're the closest we've ever come to an interventional treatment.

With time, we hope to better understand how to use these and other therapies so that the immune system will tolerate a food allergen. The benefit to you? You might be able to eat a certain food without risk of having an allergic reaction. There's also active research on interventions that might prevent food allergies from occurring in the first place. And while food intolerances aren't being researched as heavily as food allergies, there are some advances worth noting.

In this chapter, we'll look at a number of these emerging therapies and map out a possible future for food-sensitivity treatment.

Shedding Light on Food Intolerances

We know so little about many food intolerances that we certainly hope research in the future will unlock many of the mysteries and answer some of our most pressing questions. Questions that top our wish-we-knew list include the following: What causes certain food intolerances? What makes some people more prone to getting them than others? Might there be better diagnostic tools for food intolerances? Can food intolerances be treated to the point that you can actually eat the food you can't tolerate? We hope that research over the next few decades will provide some answers.

Of all of the food intolerances we've identified in this book, though, the one that is receiving a good deal of attention in the research arena is celiac disease. Currently, there's a lot of excitement about therapies that are targeting gluten and evaluating how the immune system responds to gluten. The upshot? If you have celiac disease, you might someday not have to follow such strict dietary restrictions.

Here's a sneak peek at some of these possible treatments:

- Genetically modified wheat: Researchers are currently studying whether it may be possible to grow a certain type of wheat that doesn't contain disease-causing components, making it safe for celiac patients to eat.
- Pretreated flour: Could celiac patients really eat flour? It could happen if the wheat were treated with good bacteria or pretreated with certain

enzymes, both of which would destroy disease-causing components.

- Oral enzyme therapy: An enzyme, much like those used by people who have lactose or sucrose intolerance, would be taken with food so that celiac patients could safely eat gluten.

- Neutralizing gluten antibodies: Orally ingested IgG is highly resistant to stomach acid. As a result, the IgG could reach the gut, where it may possibly neutralize gluten.

- Pharmacologic agents: Certain pharmacologic agents have been developed to increase the integrity of the intestinal lining, which might prevent gluten from crossing the intestine and triggering immune reactions.

- Immune modulators: This therapy works to inhibit certain cells in the body so that the body's immune reaction to gluten is reduced, therefore preventing damage to the intestines.

- Vaccination: A gluten vaccine has been developed to help the immune system respond differently to gluten so that when gluten is ingested, the body tolerates it. However, this therapy probably won't be available for another eight to ten years.

- Inhibition of immune cell functions: Trials are under way using small molecules to block the movement of lymphocytes to the intestine, thus eliminating immune reactions to gluten.

Advances in Food Allergies

For people with food allergies, the future is indeed bright. Several exciting therapies for food allergy are currently in various stages of development and could be just a few years away from being approved. While some of them are allergen-specific, meaning they treat only one allergen, others are not allergen specific and treat multiple food allergies at a time.

Some of these therapies have actually begun creeping into physicians' offices. However, because they haven't been thoroughly tested and no standardized protocols have been approved, we recommend waiting to try them. These therapies are still in experimental stages, which means doctors aren't exactly sure about the right treatment protocol, and there may be risks like unexpected allergic reactions and perhaps even unknown longer-term effects.

So what are some of these treatments? Let's take a look at what's in the pipeline.

Future Therapies for Immediate Food Allergies

Immunotherapy

When you have a food allergy, your immune system has gone haywire. For reasons we still don't understand, your immune system decides to attack certain food proteins that are ordinarily harmless. Yet through a treatment called immunotherapy, your immune system is retrained so it no longer views these proteins as harmful. By gradually increasing your exposure to these allergens, your body's tolerance to an allergen is increased. If all goes well, you might be able to eat your trigger food without your immune system sounding any alarm bells.

Several years ago, researchers tried treating food allergies with allergy shots, which are a form of immunotherapy. If you have an environmental allergy like a pollen or grass allergy, you're probably familiar with allergy shots, which are designed to desensitize your immune system to specific allergens. They've been fairly successful with environmental allergies. However, they failed miserably with peanut allergies because they caused too many severe, adverse reactions when used to treat them. As a result, research into food allergy shots has stopped.

Fortunately, though, other forms of immunotherapy, especially two in particular, are showing greater promise. Oral immunotherapy is one of these forms. With this therapy, you eat your allergen in gradually increasing doses. Another type of immunotherapy called sublingual treatment is similar, except that instead of swallowing large amounts of your allergen where it's mostly absorbed by the gastrointestinal tract, you place a smaller amount of your allergen, usually in the form of a drop, under your tongue, where it's primarily absorbed by your mouth's blood supply.

Both oral and sublingual immunotherapy have been tested with peanut, milk, and egg allergies and have shown good results. Success rates, meaning that study subjects are able to ingest larger amounts of allergens without reacting, generally range from 50 percent to 90 percent. Yet while it appears that both types of immunotherapy may offer some protection against accidental reactions to many food-allergic individuals, there are some pros and cons: Although sublingual immunotherapy causes fewer reactions, it isn't as protective as oral immunotherapy.

Because of those factors, researchers are now investigating whether the two therapies might be combined. The goal is to start with sublingual immunotherapy and then move to oral immunotherapy. Trials to test this combination approach have yet to begin.

Currently, though, there's a strong push to bring

oral and sublingual immunotherapy to consumers, which is why these may be one of the first advances widely available for treating immediate food allergies. In fact, some physicians are using these therapies off-label and treating patients with them, but, because the optimal dose and timing aren't known and there is considerable risk involved, we agree with most people in the field, as reflected by recent consensus guidelines sponsored by the National Institutes of Health: This therapy is not yet ready for routine clinical use.

Researchers are also experimenting with adding adjuvants, or special synthetic molecules, to food allergens. These adjuvants send strong signals to the immune system to induce a nonallergic response. Given in low doses, they might modify the allergen enough that it would be safe for food-allergic individuals to consume. So far, studies using adjuvants in people with hay fever have shown modest success, but they have yet to be tested in people with food allergies.

In addition, peptide immunotherapy is being evaluated for food allergies. A peptide is a small fragment of the food protein. Because the peptide isn't the complete protein, the theory is that when injected into the body, the peptide would not bind to IgE. As a result, no allergic reaction would occur. Although this therapy has shown positive results in people with cat allergies, it has yet to be tested in people with food allergies.

Researchers are even looking at a treatment called DNA immunization. If you're a *CSI* or *Law and Order* fan, you know DNA is the building block for your individual genetic makeup. It's what makes you, well, you.

With this therapy, researchers are hoping that by building new DNA that's coded for specific allergen proteins and injecting it in you, your immune system will recognize the DNA and produce the allergenic protein. When this happens, the hope is that your immune system would no longer see the allergen as an invader. Because your immune system would have no reason to attack the allergen, your food allergy would essentially be eliminated. While DNA immunization has shown success in diminishing peanut allergies in mice, it's still years away from being tested in humans.

Finally, another treatment involving a type of heat-treated bacteria is close to human trials. In this therapy, researchers engineer a certain type of E. coli, bacteria that are normal inhabitants of your gut, to make peanut allergens. The E. coli and peanut protein is administered through a suppository so that your immune system is exposed to the peanut protein in the presence of normal, healthy bacteria, which, like the adjuvant approach above, researchers hope will induce a protective immune response. In animal studies, the therapy has been shown to reduce or eliminate reactions. Researchers are hoping people will respond the same way.

Anti-IgE Antibody Therapy

Remember our friend IgE from chapter 6? A quick refresher: IgE is an antibody that binds to the surface of mast cells and basophils. When that IgE comes in contact with the right allergen, it triggers an allergic reaction. Keeping that in mind, researchers have developed a treatment called anti-IgE antibody therapy, which is currently being used to treat allergic asthma in kids and adults. Here's how it would work for food-allergic individuals.

Genetically engineered IgG is injected into the body. This IgG binds with IgE, rendering the IgE incapable of binding with mast cells and basophils. As a result, histamine can't be released, and there is no allergic reaction.

This therapy has already been tested in people with peanut allergies. One study found that anti-IgE antibody therapy by itself raised the average amount of peanuts needed to trigger an allergic reaction from about half a peanut to almost nine peanuts. However, one quarter of the study participants didn't benefit at all. Anti-IgE is also being used in studies with oral immunotherapy, and in one study of milk allergic individuals, it reduced reactions and allowed for more rapid therapy.

Traditional Chinese Medicine

The same herbal remedies that have been used for centuries in Asia could prove beneficial for people with immediate food allergies. Early studies have found that herbal remedies appear to be safe and may lower IgE levels for several weeks after therapy. We don't fully understand how herbal remedies work, but we suspect they somehow suppress the immune system. Studies to test whether this works in humans to prevent reactions or to alter sensitivity are ongoing.

TSO (*Trichuris Suis Ova*)

This might be the strangest sounding treatment, especially when you hear what it is. But some believe it could be an effective treatment for food allergies.

Trichuris suis ova, or TSO for short, are the eggs of a parasitic worm that naturally infects pigs. They've been tested to treat some gastrointestinal inflammatory diseases like Crohn's disease and ulcerative colitis. So how might they work for food allergies? To answer that question, take a quick trip back to chapter 3, where we discussed the hygiene hypothesis, which many experts believe is fueling the rise of food allergies. TSO works off that hypothesis.

Decades ago, our bodies were exposed to more bacteria, viruses, and parasites, all of which gave our immune system a job. Because our immune system had to spend so much time and attention on those bacteria, viruses, and parasites, it had little time to attack harmless food proteins. Meanwhile, it's been observed that people with parasitic worms have low rates of allergic diseases, which got researchers thinking: Why not introduce some of those parasites back into the body by mixing microscopic TSO eggs in a vial with water or juice and asking you to swig the liquid concoction? With TSO in your body, your immune system might be distracted enough that it stops paying attention to harmless food proteins, thus alleviating symptoms of food allergies.

The treatment is currently being explored with peanut-allergic individuals. However, it's not clear if exposing people to these noninfectious worms will provoke the same protective immune response as infectious worms do.

Probiotics

If you've got food allergies, you may someday want to order some bacteria with your next meal. Probiotics, which have been making media headlines in recent years, are live bacteria that may boost your health by balancing bacteria in your gut. Although a huge variety of bacterial species lives in your gut, researchers categorize them into two types—friendly and not-so-friendly bacteria—and believe that some diseases occur when the balance of friendly bacteria in your intestines becomes disturbed. As a result, your likelihood of having intestinal issues increases.

When you introduce probiotics into your body, though, either through supplements or foods like yogurt or kefir, the friendly bacteria displace disease-causing organisms. Balance in your intestines is thus reestablished, or so the theory goes.

In the case of food allergies, probiotics may decrease the immune system's responses to allergens. So far, though, studies have not definitely shown that probiotics can either prevent or treat food allergies.

Future Therapies for Delayed Food Allergies

Although researchers are looking at ways to prevent and treat all types of delayed food allergies, the most promising research at this point is for eosinophilic esophagitis (EoE). Below are four new therapies that might someday aid individuals who suffer from this condition.

Anti-interleukin 5 (anti-IL-5)

Interleukin-5 (IL-5) is a protein molecule that eosinophils need to survive and function. (As you'll remember from chapter 5, eosinophils are white blood cells that contribute to delayed allergic reactions.) Researchers are hoping that a drug called anti-IL-5 will reduce the survival of eosinophils, decrease the number of eosinophils in the esophagus, and inhibit their function. Two anti-IL-5 antibodies are now under investigation. Early studies have shown that anti-IL-5 reduces eosinophil numbers but does not have a significant effect on symptoms. However, future studies may perhaps identify certain individuals who would benefit.

Anti-interleukin 13 (anti-IL-13)

Interleukin-13 is an important cytokine (a protein in the body that interacts with cells of the immune system to help regulate the body's response to disease and infection) in allergic immune responses. IL-13 is thought to play a strong role in driving EoE inflammation. Currently, anti-IL-13 antibodies are being examined in hopes that they might reduce inflammatory responses in patients with EoE.

Anti-IgE

Although IgE may not have a leading role in EoE, it may play some part in causing inflammatory responses in some individuals. Anti-IgE is currently being evaluated to determine if it reduces the inflammatory responses in EoE.

Prostaglandin D2 receptor

Clinical trials are under way to target the prostaglandin D2 receptor, a hormonelike substance in the body produced by mast cells, which might decrease inflammatory responses in EoE.

Preventing Food Allergies—
Is It Possible?

Doctors can tell you how to prevent heart disease, type 2 diabetes, arthritis, even colds and the flu to some extent. Yet when it comes to preventing food allergies, research has only started to reveal some preventive strategies. While we have a long way to go before we can issue blanket recommendations for preventing food allergies, here's what we do know.

For starters, some studies have found that breast-feeding reduces the incidence of allergic disease in general, not just food allergies. A summary of studies from the journal *Pediatrics* concluded that breast-feeding for at least four months decreases the risk of allergy, especially cow's milk allergy, in a child's first two years of life, but other studies have failed to show a benefit.

Know that if you decide to breast-feed, to the best of our knowledge, you won't be increasing the chance of food allergy. The 2010 guidelines from the National Institute of Allergy and Infectious Diseases say that, although there isn't strong evidence that breast-feeding can lower your child's risk of allergy, exclusive breast-feeding for four to six months is still recommended because of the numerous other benefits it offers.

You've probably also heard you shouldn't eat peanuts while you're pregnant or else you could boost your child's risk of developing a food allergy. In fact, until recently, various key organizations supported this statement. While studies have found an association between a woman's consumption of peanuts during pregnancy and increased levels of IgE in her child, keep in mind a few important points, which will help you understand why guidelines have recently shifted.

First, having increased levels of IgE doesn't necessarily mean a child will develop a clinical allergy to that food. Second, researchers can't say with any certainty that the mother's consumption of peanuts raised her child's risk. The child's exposure to peanuts could have come from anywhere in the environment. Finally, studies of early infant ingestion have found the opposite to be true, too. Consistent with this, the National Institute of Allergy and Infectious Diseases doesn't recommend that women make any dietary restrictions during lactation, including for "high-risk" children, and we agree.

Another possible preventive strategy? Food introduction. We no longer believe that delaying solid foods, especially those known to cause food allergies, is wise. The American Academy of Pediatrics now recommends introducing solid foods when children are between four and six months old.

Those recommendations, by the way, also apply to high-risk children, or those who have a genetic predisposition to allergies, including siblings of children who have a known food allergy. There's no evidence that waiting to introduce foods to their diet is helpful. In fact, delaying foods could wind up causing more problems.

Here's what all of this boils down to: You shouldn't blame yourself if your child develops a food allergy. Given what we currently know, preventing allergies of

Apps for Food Sensitivities

Your doctor isn't the only one who can help you manage your food sensitivity. Turns out, your smartphone could come in handy, too. We looked at dozens of apps on the market and thought these eight were worth mentioning:

- **Allergy Passport** (www.pistolshrimp.mobi/AllergyPassport/): Traveling just got easier thanks to this app, which asks you to identify your food allergies, choose the language you want to convey your message in, and select your message. The translation pops up on your screen so you can pass it to your waiter, dinner host, or chef.
- **CookItAllergyFree** (www.cookitallergyfree.com): This app, which was created by a woman who holds a master's degree in nutrition and is the mother of a son with celiac disease, features hundreds of gluten-free recipes that can be customized for any food allergy. You can also find substitutions for the most common trigger foods and tips for allergy-free cooking.
- **EMNet findER** (http://itunes.apple.com/app/emnet-finder/id376928203?mt=8): Locate the nearest emergency room with just one click in this app from Massachusetts General Hospital.

- **iCanEatOnTheGo** (www.allergyfreepassport.com): Explore twenty menus from leading chain restaurants in the United States and see which of two thousand items contains any combination of the following trigger foods: eggs, fish, gluten, milk, peanuts, shellfish, soy, tree nuts, and wheat.

- **Is That Gluten Free? Eating Out** (http://midlifecrisisapps .com/): Not sure which restaurant offers gluten-free meals? With this app, you can scan through national and regional restaurant chains for gluten-free options.

- **Is That Gluten Free? for Groceries** (http://midlifecrisis apps.com/): Take this app to the grocery store, and you'll be able to scroll through a list of over fifty brands to identify gluten-free items.

- **MyEpiPenApp** (www.epipen.com/about-the-myepipen app): With this app from EpiPen, you can show others how to use an EpiPen and create allergy profiles of your family members that can be shared.

- **MyFoodFacts** (www.myfoodfacts.com): Scan the UPC bar code of a particular food at the grocery store, and this app will search for food allergens and alert you if it finds anything suspicious about that food.

Want to help shape the future of food sensitivities? Become a study subject

If you want to play a role in helping uncover new facts about food sensitivities, you don't need to go to medical school to get a degree. Just sign up for a clinical research study. While there isn't any financial reward, you'll have the satisfaction of helping advance our knowledge of food sensitivities, which could someday lead to more effective treatments and potential cures.

To locate studies, ask your primary care physician, allergist, or gastroenterologist if they've heard of any studies recruiting people with food allergies. You can also check federally and privately supported clinical trials by logging on to www.clinicaltrials.gov. Or, log on to the Web site of the American Academy of Allergy, Asthma and Immunology (www.aaaai.org), which often announces studies that are actively seeking individuals.

any kind, especially food allergies, is impossible. Theoretically, if your child were never exposed to any allergen, no allergy would develop. Yet in the real world, that's not possible. Allergens are present everywhere in the environment, and it's impossible to escape them.

Take, for instance, cat and peanut allergens. Both allergens have shown up in surprising places: For cat allergens, in homes of people who have never owned a cat, and for peanut allergens, in dust samples taken from public places.

Whether they're in the air we breathe or the food we eat, allergens are simply part of our environment. While we can never escape them, we hope that in the near future, we can learn to coexist with them better.

acknowledgments

This book wouldn't have been possible without the help of these individuals:

Julie Silver, MD, chief editor in books at Harvard Health Publications, who put our team together and helped shape the book's concept. We appreciate your encouragement and guidance.

Linda Konner, our literary agent.

Meredith Mennitt, our editor at St. Martin's, who made the whole process seamless—and our words that much more effective.

Finally, Wayne and Qian would like to thank our patients, who always have something new to teach us.

resources and references

If you'd like to learn more about food intolerances and food allergies, we recommend that you check out the following resources.

Associations and Foundations
Academy of Nutrition and Dietetics
120 South Riverside Plaza, Suite 2000
Chicago, IL 60606-6995
800-877-1600
www.eatright.org

American Academy of Allergy, Asthma and Immunology
555 East Wells Street, Suite 1100
Milwaukee, WI 53202-3823
414-272-6071
www.aaaai.org

American Academy of Pediatrics
141 Northwest Point Boulevard
Elk Grove Village, IL 60007-1098
847-434-4000
www.aap.org

American Celiac Disease Alliance
2504 Duxbury Place
Alexandria, VA 22308
703-622-3331
www.americanceliac.org

American Celiac Society Dietary Support Coalition
P.O. Box 23455
New Orleans, LA 70183
504-737-3293
www.americanceliacsociety.org

American College of Allergy, Asthma and Immunology
85 West Algonquin Road, Suite 550
Arlington Heights, IL 60005
847-427-1200
www.acaai.org

American Gastroenterological Association
4930 Del Ray Avenue
Bethesda, MD 20814
301-654-2055
www.gastro.org

American Partnership for Eosinophilic Disorders
P.O. Box 29545

Atlanta, GA 30359
713-493-7749
www.apfed.org

Association of Pediatric Gastroenterology
and Nutrition Nurses
P.O. Box 6
Flourtown, PA 19031
215-233-0808
www.apgnn.org

Asthma and Allergy Foundation of America
8201 Corporate Drive, Suite 1000
Landover, MD 20785
800-7-ASTHMA
www.aafa.org

Celiac Disease Foundation
13251 Ventura Boulevard, Suite 1
Studio City, CA 91604
818-990-2354
www.celiac.org

Celiac Sprue Association
P.O. Box 31700
Omaha, NE 68131-0700

877-CSA-4CSA
www.csaceliacs.info

Children's Digestive Health and
Nutrition Foundation
P.O. Box 6
Flourtown, PA 19031
215-233-0808
www.cdhnf.org

Food Allergy and Anaphylaxis Network
11781 Lee Jackson Highway, Suite 160
Fairfax, VA 22033-3309
800-929-4040
www.foodallergy.org

Food Allergy Initiative
515 Madison Avenue, Suite 1912
New York, NY 10022-5403
855-FAI-9604
212-207-1974
www.faiusa.org

Gluten Intolerance Group of North America
31214 124th Avenue SE
Auburn, WA 98092-3667

253-833-6655
www.gluten.net

International Gastrointestinal Eosinophil
Researchers (TIGER)
http://tiger-egid.cdhnf.org

National Foundation for Celiac Awareness
224 South Maple Street
Ambler, PA 19002
215-325-1306
www.celiaccentral.org

National Institute of Allergy and Infectious Diseases
National Institutes of Health
6610 Rockledge Drive, MSC 6612
Bethesda, MD 20892-6612
866-284-4107
www.niaid.nih.gov

North American Society for Pediatric Gastroenterology,
Hepatology and Nutrition
P.O. Box 6
Flourtown, PA 19031
215-233-0808
www.naspghan.org

Books

Understanding and Managing Your Child's Food Allergies, by Scott H. Sicherer, M.D. (Johns Hopkins University Press, 2006)

Web Sites

The Consortium for Food Allergy Research
www.cofar.org

Food allergy guidelines from the National Institute of Allergy and Infectious Diseases
http://www.niaid.nih.gov

Kids with Food Allergies Foundation
www.kidswithfoodallergies.org

notes

1: Learning the Lingo

See http://www.bartleby.com/100/703.html.

See http://www.gastro.org/patient-center/diet-medications/food -allergies-fructose-intolerance-and-lactose-intolerance.

See http://www.cdc.gov/media/pressrel/2008/r081022.htm.

2: Who's Most at Risk for Developing a Food Sensitivity?

M. H. K. Ho, S. Lee, W. H. S. Wong, Y. Lau. (2010). "Peanut Oil and Peanut Allergy, Foes or Folks?" *Archives of Disease in Childhood* 95: 856–57.

See http://www.aaaai.org/patients/advocate/2006/spring/child_ allergist.asp.

S. H. Sicherer, T. J. Furlong, H. H. Maes, R. J. Desnick, H. A. Sampson, B. D. Gelb. (2000). "Genetics of Peanut Allergy: A Twin Study." *Journal of Allergy and Clinical Immunology* 106: 53–56.

See http://digestive.niddk.nih.gov/ddiseases/pubs/celiac/#diag nosis.

I. Smidesang, M. Saunes, O. Storrø, T. Øien, T. L. Holmen, R. Johnsen, and A. H. Henriksen. (2010). "Allergy Related Disorders Among 2-Yrs Olds in a General Population." "The PACT Study." *Pediatric Allergy and Immunology* 21: 315–20.

See http://www.cdhnf.org/user-assets/documents/pdf/A%20 Guide%20to%20Eosinophilic%20Esophagitis%20in% 20Children%20and%20Adults.pdf.

3: Are Food Sensitivities on the Rise?

See http://digestive.niddk.nih.gov/ddiseases/pubs/ibs/.

See http://www.packagedfacts.com/about/release.asp?id=1864.

See http://www.cdc.gov/healthyyouth/foodallergies/.

See http://www.cdc.gov/nchs/data/databriefs/db10.htm.

R. S. Gupta, E. E. Springston, M. R. Warrier, B. Smith, R. Kumar, J. Pongracic, J. L. Holl. (2011). "The Prevalence, Severity, and Distribution of Childhood Food Allergy in the United States." *Pediatrics* 10.1542/peds.2011-0204.

Roberto J. Rona, Thomas Keil, Colin Summers, David Gislason, Laurian Zuidmeer, Eva Sodergren, Sigurveig T. Sigurdardottir, Titia Lindner, Klaus Goldhahn, Jorgen Dahlstrom, Doreen McBride, Charlotte Madsen. (2007). "The Prevalence of Food Allergy: A Meta-analysis." *Journal of Allergy and Clinical Immunology* 120(3): 638–46.

Jennifer J. Schneider Chafen, Sydne J. Newberry, Marc A. Riedl, Dena M. Bravata, Margaret Maglione, Marika J. Suttorp, Vandana Sundaram, Neil M. Paige, Ali Towfigh, Benjamin J. Hulley, Paul G. Shekelle. (2010). "Diagnosing and Managing Common Food Allergies: A Systematic Review." *Journal of the American Medical Association* 303(18): 1848–56.

B. J. Vlieg-Boerstra, S. Van Der Heide, C. M. A. Bijleveld, J. Kukler, E. J. Duiverman, and A. E. J. Dubois. (2007). "Placebo Reactions in Double-Blind, Placebo-Controlled Food Challenges in Children." *Allergy* 62: 905–12.

See http://www.cdc.gov/media/pressrel/2008/r081022.htm.

M. H. K. Ho, S. Lee, W. H. S. Wong, Y. Lau. (2010). "Peanut Oil and Peanut Allergy, Foes or Folks?" *Archives of Disease in Childhood* 95: 856–57.

C. A. Camargo, S. Clark, J. F. Pearson, M. S. Kaplan, P. Lieberman, R. A. Wood. (2009). "Latitude, UVB Exposure, and EpiPen Prescriptions in 38 Urban Areas." *Journal of Allergy and Clinical Immunology* 123(2): S109.

See http://visitbakersfield.com/media/facts/.

See http://www.bellingham.org/discover/climate/.

G. Du Toit, Y. Katz, P. Sasieni, D. Mesher, S. J. Maleki, H. R. Fisher, A. T. Fox, V. Turcanu, T. Amir, G. Zadik-Mnuhin,

A. Cohen, I. Livne, G. Lack. (2008). "Early Consumption of
Peanuts in Infancy Is Associated with a Low Prevalence of
Peanut Allergy." *Journal of Allergy and Clinical Immunology*
122(5): 984–91.

Yitzhak Katz, Nelly Rajuan, Michael R. Goldberg, Eli Eisen-
berg, Eli Heyman, Adi Cohen, Moshe Leshno. (2010). "Early
Exposure to Cow's Milk Protein Is Protective Against IgE-
Mediated Cow's Milk Protein Allergy." *Journal of Allergy and
Clinical Immunology* 126(1): 77–82.e1.

Jennifer J. Koplin, Nicholas J. Osborne, Melissa Wake, Pamela
E. Martin, Lyle C. Gurrin, Marnie N. Robinson, Dean
Tey, Marjolein Slaa, Leone Thiele, Lucy Miles, Deborah
Anderson, Tina Tan, Thanh D. Dang, David J. Hill, Adrian J.
Lowe, Melanie C. Matheson, Anne-Louise Ponsonby, Mimi
L. K. Tang, Shyamali C. Dharmage, Katrina J. Allen. (2010).
"Can Early Introduction of Egg Prevent Egg Allergy in In-
fants? A Population-Based Study." *Journal of Allergy and Clini-
cal Immunology* 126(4): 807–13.

4: Food Intolerances 101

A. O. Johnson, J. G. Semenya, S. M. Buchowski, C. O. En-
wonwu, and N. S. Scrimshaw. (1993). "Correlation of Lactose
Maldigestion, Lactose Intolerance, and Milk Intolerance."
American Journal of Clinical Nutrition 57(3): 399–401.

See www.uptodate.com/contents/patient-information-celiac
-disease-in-adults.

5: Getting a Handle on Common Intolerances

See http://www.nichd.nih.gov/publications/pubs/upload/NIC
HD_MM_Lactose_FS.pdf.

See http://www.gastro.org/patient-center/diet-medications/food
-allergies-fructose-intolerance-and-lactose-intolerance.

See http://ods.od.nih.gov/factsheets/calcium/.

See http://www.iom.edu/Reports/2010/Dietary-Reference-In
takes-for-Calcium-and-Vitamin-D/DRI-Values.aspx.

See http://ods.od.nih.gov/factsheets/vitamind/.

See http://nutritiondata.self.com/foods-0000110000000000
   00000.html.

C. Catassi, D. Kryszak, B. Bhatti, C. Sturgeon, K. Helzlsouer,
   S. L. Clipp, D. Gelfond, E. Puppa, A. Sferruzza, A. Fasano.
   (2010). "National History of Celiac Disease Autoimmunity
   in a USA Cohort Followed Since 1974." *Annals of Medicine*
   42(7): 530–38.

See http://www.celiac.org/images/stories/PDF/general-brochure
   -2010.pdf.

See http://www.celiac.org/images/stories/PDF/are-you-the-one
   .pdf.

See http://www.celiac.org/images/stories/PDF/general-brochure
   -2010.pdf.

6: Let's Evaluate Your Symptoms

Sunday Clark, Janice Espinola, Susan A. Rudders, Aleena Ba-
   nerji, Carlos A. Camargo. (2010). "Frequency of US Emergency Department Visits for Food-Related Acute Allergic
   Reactions." *Journal of Allergy and Clinical Immunology* 127(3):
   682–83.

See http://www.cdc.gov/healthyyouth/foodallergies/.

These are estimates. See http://www.cdc.gov/nchs/data/data
   briefs/db10.pdf and http://www.niaid.nih.gov/topics/food
   Allergy/clinical/Documents/FAguidelinesPatient.pdf.

See http://www.cdc.gov/healthyyouth/foodallergies/.

See http://www.aaaai.org/media/statistics/allergy-statistics.asp.

Scott H. Sicherer, Anne Muñoz-Furlong, James H. Godbold, Hugh
   A. Sampson. (2010). "US Prevalence of Self-reported Peanut,
   Tree Nut, and Sesame Allergy: 11-Year Follow-up." *Journal of
   Allergy and Clinical Immunology* 125(6): 1322–26.

See http://www.aaaai.org/media/statistics/allergy-statistics.asp.

See http://www.faiusa.org/page.aspx?pid=362.

S. J. Simonte, S. Ma, S. Mofidi, S. H. Sicherer. (2003). "Relevance
   of Casual Contact with Peanut Butter in Children with Peanut
   Allergy." *Journal of Allergy and Clinical Immunology* 112(1):
   180–82.

See http://www.aaaai.org/media/statistics/allergy-statistics.asp.
See http://www.foodallergy.org/page/other.
See http://www.cdhnf.org/user-assets/documents/pdf/A%20
    Guide%20to%20Eosinophilic%20Esophagitis%20in%
    20Children%20and%20Adults.pdf.

7: The Doctor Will See You Now

See http://nccam.nih.gov/health/whatiscam/.

8: Living with Food Allergies

See www.med.umich.edu/mott/npch/reports/foodallergy.htm.
See http://www.foodallergy.org/page/airport-security.

9: Will There Ever Be a Cure for Food Sensitivities?

Donald Y. M. Leung, Hugh A. Sampson, John W. Yunginger, A.
    Wesley Burks, Jr., Lynda C. Schneider, Cornelis H. Wortel,
    Frances M. Davis, John D. Hyun, B.S., and William R. Sha-
    nahan, Jr. (2003). "Effect of Anti-IgE Therapy in Patients
    with Peanut Allergy." *New England Journal of Medicine* 348:
    986–93.
Frank R. Greer, Scott H. Sicherer, A. Wesley Burks, and the
    Committee on Nutrition and Section on Allergy and Immu-
    nology. (2008). "Effects of Early Nutritional Interventions
    on the Development of Atopic Disease in Infants and Chil-
    dren: The Role of Maternal Dietary Restriction, Breastfeed-
    ing, Timing of Introduction of Complementary Foods, and
    Hydrolyzed Formulas." *Pediatrics* 121(1): 183–91.
See http://www.niaid.nih.gov/topics/foodAllergy/understanding/
    Pages/Pregnancy.aspx.

Index

From Harvard Health Publications...
Trusted Advice for a *healthier* Life

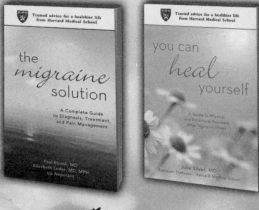

ST. MARTIN'S GRIFFIN